ACTUARIALLY DETERMINED CAPITATION RATES FOR MENTAL HEALTH BENEFITS

Report Prepared for the American Psychiatric Association

Stephen P. Melek, FSA, MAAA
Bruce S. Pyenson, FSA, MAAA

September 21, 1995

Prepared by MILLIMAN & ROBERTSON, INC.,
Actuaries and Consultants, New York, New York

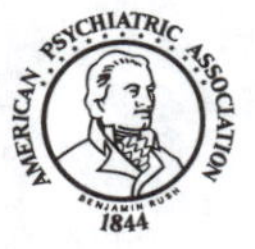

American Psychiatric Association
1400 K Street, NW
Washington, DC 20005

Contents

About the Authors

STEPHEN P. MELEK, FSA, MAAA
Consulting Actuary

Steve is a Consulting Actuary with the Denver office of Milliman & Robertson, Inc. His areas of expertise include healthcare product development, management, and financial analysis, with a particular emphasis in behavioral healthcare. He has experience with plan design, pricing, capitation analysis and development, risk analysis, reimbursement analysis and strategies, healthcare revenue distribution and utilization management analysis. Additionally, Steve has experience with valuations and projections of healthcare businesses, profitability and experience analysis, reinsurance, pricing models and strategies and actuarial liability determinations. Steve has advised hospitals, physician groups, PHOs, HMOs, PPOs, managed care organizations, behavioral healthcare firms and associations, insurance companies, employers and state insurance departments.

BRUCE S. PYENSON, FSA, MAAA
Consulting Actuary

Bruce is a Consulting Actuary with the New York City office of Milliman & Robertson, Inc. He consults to management in a wide range of managed care organizations, insurers, employers, and healthcare providers and suppliers on issues ranging from market strategies and capitation development to healthcare reform. His time with Milliman & Robertson includes a year spent in the United Kingdom where he consulted to the growing private healthcare sector. Bruce, a Fellow of the Society of Actuaries and a Member of the American Academy of Actuaries, is the editor and co-author of *Calculated Risk: A Provider's Guide to Assessing and Controlling the Financial Risk of Managed Care* (American Hospital Publishing, 1995). He is also the co-author of *Employee Benefits for Small Business* (JK Lasser, Simon & Schuster, 1991, 1992). Bruce is a frequent speaker at industry gatherings.

A Note From the President of the American Psychiatric Association

This much awaited *American Psychiatric Association Capitation Handbook* is a product in keeping with the overarching goals that I identified at the 1995 Fall Leadership Conference. It represents the united effort of the APA leadership; actuarial consultants at Milliman & Robertson, Inc., knowledgeable experts in the field; the Committee on Managed Care, chaired by Jeremy A. Lazarus, M.D.; the Council on Economic Affairs, which was chaired by Paul J. Fink, M.D., and which is now chaired by William Goldman, M.D.; and the Office of Economic Affairs.

This study will serve as a guide for our members and for nonmembers who are entering capitated agreements. Capitation rates that are too low or inadequate may impede access to appropriate treatment.

I hope that by providing guidance and information on capitation, capitation rates, and how various factors affect capitation rates under different scenarios and for different populations, this study will eventually improve access to appropriate care, especially for vulnerable populations.

Mary Jane England, M.D.

A NOTE FROM JEREMY A. LAZARUS, M.D.

It is with great pleasure that the American Psychiatric Association (APA) is providing the enclosed study on capitation commissioned by the APA. This document is the end result of an action in the Assembly of the APA that asked that the APA advocate for adequate funding in capitation contracts for the mentally ill. While the APA does not specifically advocate for the use of capitation, it is clear that there are increasing numbers of managed care contracts that are negotiated under capitation. The APA has been quite concerned that certain very low capitations will not allow adequate access or treatment for the mentally ill. While there are numerous pitfalls in contracting under capitation, the first part of this report outlines the major areas to be aware of in the process. Of concern to us all was that there should be adequate capitation to provide for the reasonable treatment of the mentally ill. In the enclosed charts it is possible to determine the actual numbers of services that can be provided under various scenarios and thereby whether the care can be considered adequate.

The approach that the Committee on Managed Care, Council on Economic Affairs, and Board eventually took was to ask a well-known actuarial firm to develop comprehensive capitation scenarios for the commercial and Medicare populations. In addition, we authorized development of capitation scenarios for a national average for Medicaid with the recognition that there are numerous factors influencing individual state Medicaid capitations. This would have expanded our project well beyond our financial capabilities.

The comprehensive commercial charts serve as a template on which psychiatric providers can gauge the real numbers of services they can provide with defined variables such as discount, amount of management of care, and geographic payment averages. These charts cannot be used alone for contracting purposes, and members are advised to get appropriate advice prior to negotiating for capitated contracts.

This document was reviewed by members of the Committee on Managed Care, Council on Economic Affairs, and Board. Many from those components with broad knowledge of capitation made invaluable contributions during the drafting of the document. My special thanks to Paul Fink, M.D., and Henry Harbin, M.D., without whose help this document could not have been easily completed. Finally, my thanks to Steve Melek and Bruce Pyenson from Milliman & Robertson, who worked closely with me in drafting and redrafting the document so that it would reflect the values and concerns of the APA.

Jeremy A. Lazarus, M.D.
Chair, Committee on Managed Care

I. EXECUTIVE SUMMARY

The American Psychiatric Association (APA) commissioned Milliman & Robertson, Inc. (M&R), to prepare this report on capitation rates for alcohol, drug and mental disease (ADM) services. The purpose of this report is to provide general guidance and education to APA members on capitation, capitation rates and how various factors may affect such rates. This report may not be suitable for other purposes.

In recent years, specialty capitation programs have expanded rapidly. Many HMOs, insurers and health plans capitate ADM services. These programs may operate through mental health carve-out companies, through integrated delivery systems, or through individual or group mental health practices. Capitated programs may cover the commercial population, Medicare eligibles or the Medicaid populations. The capitation rates paid vary widely, as do the definitions of covered services, managed care practices, and local cost levels. The APA commissioned this report to provide its members with guidance in how and why capitation rates may vary.

The marketplace determines, to a large extent, prices in the healthcare system. To a large extent, the market determines the premium rates that insurers and HMOs can charge, and the fees and capitation rates they must pay. Capitation rates, as any new commodity, may sometimes reflect some of the chaos of the market—and naiveté of the buyer or provider—and be either too high or too low. There may be no real relationship between a carefully devised capitation rate and one that a particular market will bear. But developing a base rate will help providers to develop a range of services for a price that the market will shoulder.

Fees and capitation rates also usually reflect underlying demand for services, local fee levels, patient cost sharing and the way care is handled. Actuarial analysis and data offer a window to look at the elements that go into the prices and services rendered, and to gain insight into how these elements interact. This report presents these factors and offers many examples of how they interact to produce particular capitation rates.

The American Psychiatric Association represents over 40,000 psychiatrists in the U.S. and other countries. This study was developed and coordinated by the APA's Committee on Managed Care, chaired by Jeremy Allan Lazarus, M.D., the Council on Economic Affairs, which was chaired by Paul J. Fink, M.D., and the Office of Economic Affairs.

Milliman & Robertson, Inc., almost 50 years old, is a firm of actuaries and consultants and a leading source of actuarial expertise to Blue Cross Blue Shield Plans, health insurers, HMOs and healthcare providers. Located in 25 U.S. cities and Tokyo, M&R employs over 400 actuaries with professional designations.

We developed capitation rates in this report by applying actuarial relationships among benefit limits, local costs, degree of healthcare management, patient cost sharing, and provider discounts for ADM services.

Certain combinations of these factors (e.g., low benefit plans combined with low local cost levels, aggressive care management, high patient cost sharing, and large provider discounts) produce low capitation rates. We recognize the APA's concerns that overly low capitation rates simply may not allow physicians to provide an adequate amount of care. Certainly, poor quality or poor access can occur in plans that appear to offer generous benefits or reimbursement. We do not intend for this report to be used by organizations to justify inadequate capitation rates for ADM providers. Rather, we present rates associated with these various combinations of factors in order to provide general guidance and education to APA members on these capitation issues.

This report should not be used as the basis for deciding whether or not to enter into a capitation agreement. Medical providers and others must consider many important issues beyond those reported here. Competent legal and actuarial advice should be obtained before judging any particular proposal.

In conducting and reporting on this study, Milliman & Robertson does not intend to take a position on any particular legislation. The conclusions of this study are based on the authors' analysis and should not be interpreted as representing the position of Milliman & Robertson, Inc.

II. INTRODUCTION AND QUALIFICATIONS

Milliman & Robertson, Inc. (M&R) was retained by the American Psychiatric Association (APA) to estimate the costs for alcohol, drug and mental disease (ADM) services under capitation arrangements.

This report presents the following estimates:

1. Capitation rates for ADM services for the commercial population under a variety of scenarios including various benefit designs, copays, local cost levels, managed care efforts and discounts
2. Capitation rates for ADM services for the Medicare population under a variety of scenarios including various local cost levels, managed care efforts, copays and discounts
3. Capitation rates for ADM services for the Medicaid population under a variety of cost and utilization scenarios

This report presents these cost estimates along with descriptions of the data sources, methodology and assumptions that we used to produce the cost estimates.

We also present general information about how capitation works and how behavioral healthcare providers can deal with the risks of managed care.

Because the economy and the healthcare system are dynamic, there is an intrinsic uncertainty in projecting costs for any healthcare coverage, and this uncertainty applies to our work. The estimates presented here are based on a number of assumptions, partly because data about mental health and substance abuse utilization and demand are incomplete, especially in the area of non-discriminatory behavioral benefits for the commercial population. We present cost estimates for various combinations of plan assumptions, some of which result in higher capitation rates and some in low rates. We recognize that very low capitation rates may pose problems for physicians regarding adequate quality or access. Actual costs will differ from the results presented to the extent that the actual utilization or charge levels differ from those assumed. Nevertheless, we believe that the assumptions and methodology we have used are reasonable, as are our estimates.

This report is not intended to support or detract from any particular legislation.

III. ASSUMPTIONS AND LIMITATIONS

We independently estimated the costs for three of the most important populations that are increasingly covered through capitated arrangements:

1. The insured, non-Medicare "commercial" population
2. The over-65 Medicare population
3. The Medicaid population

For each of the three populations, we used age/sex demographic assumptions consistent with national population data. Specific demographic data for any particular group will most likely differ from the national distribution, and such differences should be recognized in any specific capitation analyses.

This report follows the usual HMO and insurance industry practice of presenting estimated costs in *per-member-per-month* (PMPM) units. These costs represent the average claim cost that a member incurs in one month. The industry considers each covered life—whether child or adult—as a "member." The average member age for the commercial and Medicaid populations reflects a mix of children and adults and is generally lower than the age of the average adult. Consequently, the PMPM net claim cost for these populations is lower than the net claim cost for an adult. We do not expand the PMPM costs to show "market" units such as the cost of single or family coverage.

No explicit margins or allowances for administrative expenses, co-ordination of benefits, stop loss reinsurance, adverse risks, or margins for profits and/or contingencies beyond those implicitly provided within the average costs per unit of service have been used.

Insurers and HMOs usually include in their premium rates a margin for administrative expenses from 5% to 15% and also include additional margins for adverse risk charges, profits and/or contingencies.

The Commercial Population

The starting point for our cost estimates for the currently insured population is the M&R *Health Cost Guidelines* (HCGs) (July 1995 edition). The HCGs are M&R's proprietary information base that shows how the components of per-capita medical and behavioral claim costs vary with benefit design, demography, location, provider reimbursement arrangements, and other factors. An extensive amount of data are used in developing the HCGs. In most instances, cost assumptions are based on our evaluation of several data sources and are not specifically attributable to a single source. The HCGs are used by client insurance companies for, primarily, pricing and evaluating insured products. As such, the HCGs are not necessarily appropriate for uninsured or Medicaid populations.

We also incorporated information from the M&R *Healthcare Management Guidelines* which provides information regarding the effect of managed care principles and clinical protocols on medical and behavioral care utilization. The *Healthcare Management Guidelines* are the result of several years' efforts to develop an effective resource to manage the cost, quality, and delivery of healthcare services.

The Medicare Population

The starting point for our cost estimates for the currently insured population is the M&R Over-65 *Health Cost Guidelines* (HCGs) (July 1995 edition), which provides utilization and cost information for the Medicare aged population, including billed charge and Medicare allowed charge information. We also incorporated information from the M&R *Healthcare Management Guidelines* and from data files obtained from the Health Care Financing Administration (HCFA).

The methodology for the Medicare population is described in more detail in Section IX and Appendix II.

The Medicaid Population

We analyzed several sources of information to develop cost estimates for the Medicaid population including data from NASMHPD (Funding Sources and Expenditures of State Mental Health Agencies), available data for Medicaid populations in four states by eligibility category, published AM-BHA managed Medicaid experience, and proprietary managed behavioral healthcare data of M&R. We describe the methodology for the Medicaid population in more detail in Section X and Appendix II.

Overview of Capitation Basics

IV. CAPITATION BASICS

This section of the report presents an overview of capitation principles, applications, and the advantages and disadvantages of this type of reimbursement structure. For most providers, the risks inherent in capitation contracts have only recently emerged. Capitation payments to providers resemble the premiums that insurance companies traditionally collect. Under capitation, providers are assuming many of the risks that insurers formerly assumed. As providers become the risk-takers in the healthcare delivery system, they should consider the actuarial issues related to their individual contracts in order to understand the value of these risks and the potential opportunities afforded to them.

General Capitation Principles

Most capitation payments consist of an established monthly payment to a provider in exchange for a defined set of medical or behavioral services to an identified individual. The capitation amount varies with the services covered, the copays, and the age, sex, and other characteristics of the covered individual. Actuaries sometimes call the factors that help determine the capitation rate for an individual "risk factors." For group health insurance, group risk factors may include whether everyone in a group is actively-at-work, the employer's size, and may include certain requirements for participation or insurability.

For individual life insurance, the risk classification may be: men, ages 50–59, who do not smoke, whose HDL ratio is less than 4, whose GGT level is less than 65, and who have no history of parental heart disease. Insurers and HMOs term the process of determining the risk factors for an individual or group *underwriting*. We present capitation rates in Sections VIII through X for typical cross-sections of each of the commercially insured population, Medicare population, and Medicaid populations.

When a health plan pays capitations to a provider, the covered (or client) population for that provider consists of individuals who have chosen that provider or individuals who the health plan has assigned to that provider. The payment to the provider is, in simple terms,

♦ the number of members

    times

♦ the capitation rate

The capitation rate generally varies with the age and sex of the member, and the health plan tabulates members by age and sex categories.

Capitation transfers the insurance risk from one party (the insurer, health plan or HMO) to another party (the medical provider). Health plans have structured capitation arrangements in many ways. Capitation arrangements with healthcare providers integrate insurance risk with provider compensation; the *capitated* (provider) assumes the insurance risk for a defined scope of services, much like an insurance company. The more favorable the actual payment to the *capitated,* when compared to traditional fee-for-service reimbursement, the greater the financial benefit for the *capitated* of the capitation form of reimbursement.

While capitation payments for an individual usually occur monthly, the services that the provider actually delivers to that individual will probably occur irregularly, if at all. The uncertainty in the timing and amount of service contrasts to the certainty of the capitation payment, and this contrast generates risk for the provider. A provider faces the least risk when the demand for capitated services is relatively predictable. Consequently, physicians usually face less risk capitating primary care and preventive services than capitating rare services such as organ transplants. The predictability of certain kinds of services, or the services rendered to large numbers of people, can make capitation a good alternative to fee-for-service payment methodologies.

In practice, any given health plan may or may not limit capitation to particular types of service or grouping of services. Providers need to evaluate the risks and benefits of any given capitation proposal by considering the following issues:

♦ What are the risks?
♦ What is the financial value of these risks?
♦ What is the potential variation of these financial risks?

Sometimes an HMO or insurer will offer providers a rate for a set of benefits and the providers must decide if they can live with it. To meet this price target, providers may attempt to shuffle the types of services provided or renegotiate professional rates. That, for example, may mean using more allied professionals or using more group therapy.

Evaluating a capitation proposal usually involves translating a contract into an actuarial model like those the authors used to develop this report's estimates. This may involve calculating the fee-for-service equivalent of a given capitation rate and estimating the effects on cost of various managed care efforts. The details of this process are beyond the scope of this report.

Reasons for the Growing Interest in Capitation

In recent decades, insurers and managed care organizations have often seen their efforts to control utilization and cost yield less than hoped for results. These organizations now often see capitation as a successful way to reduce costs. The capitation rates that many health plans pay translate into a fairly steep fee-for-service discount. However, simple fee-for-service discounts have generally not yielded cost savings as great as those of capitation rates. The success of capitation stems, at least partly, from its success in bringing providers into the cost management process.

Capitation arrangements have proven attractive to many providers as well. Capitation arrangements offer the provider an incentive to reduce his or her own costs. Under capitation, a provider's cost reductions increases his or her profit, while, under fee-for-service arrangements, increased utilization usually results in greater provider profit.

Capitation follows naturally from the managed care principle of managing within a budget. Furthermore, insurers, whose income takes the form of premium payments, in effect take capitation payments from their customers. Conceptually, insurers probably grasp the concept of capitation more easily than do many medical practitioners.

Other advantages of capitation include the stability of cash flow—for both the payer and provider. Providers may prefer the stable revenue flows of capitation as a way to ease revenue uncertainty. Governments (who pay for Medicare and Medicaid and the sizable government employee programs) perceive that capitation provides stable expenditures and produces more predictable budgets. Employers also take these perspectives as they see that capitation can control costs and lead to more certain benefit costs. Some employers have incorporated capitation into their self-funded employee benefit programs. Knowledgeable payers realize that the provider, as well as the employer, can benefit from the reduced level of utilization under capitation.

From both the payer and the provider perspectives, capitation offers advantages and disadvantages, including

Payer Advantages:

♦ Transfer difficult or seemingly uncontrollable risks
♦ Minimize unexpected variations in cost
♦ Involve providers in the risk control process
♦ Manage providers effectively (providers start to manage themselves)

Payer Disadvantages:

♦ May lose some control over providers if data not captured
♦ May lose some control over members
♦ Providers might not control consumption and become dissatisfied
♦ Potentially difficult or slow negotiations
♦ Need remains for payer to monitor quality, appropriateness, and effectiveness of care

Provider Advantages:

♦ Can preserve net income while reducing number or intensity of services delivered
♦ Stabilizes revenue flows, lends itself to traditional business management approaches

- Provides a more direct link between potential patients and provider group
- Lends itself to exclusive contracting and an improved potential to preserve patient base
- Helps provider link the cost of care with their practice patterns to better understand how to manage care

Provider Disadvantages:

- Requires additional technical skills not always available in provider group
- Serious financial difficulties can result if services are not appropriately controlled
- Potential for payer to take advantage of provider by including more and more services without appropriate increases in the capitation
- Careful analysis required to determine actual value of contract
- Requires capital base for risk reserves to protect provider from statistical fluctuations
- Need an effective way to distribute funds among providers when providers are capitated
- Provider must become a mini-insurance company
- Potential for additional administrative costs

Factors Influencing Successful Capitation

V.   KEYS TO SUCCESSFUL CAPITATION

Providers and payers should have the following information as part of a capitation arrangement:

♦ A clear definition of eligible members
♦ An idea of what constitutes a sufficient volume of covered members
♦ An understanding of whether the amount of services promise will be manageable
♦ A definable scope of services
♦ A view of potential cost shifting across provider groups
♦ A plan to control consumption and/or adequate teamwork with one who does
♦ Commitment to fair negotiations by both sides over long term
♦ Reasonable links between capitated population and provider group
♦ An actuarially sound basis for adjusting capitation rates

All capitation programs should have this sort of information, but new types of programs, including behavioral healthcare specialty programs, need to understand these issues.

Clear Definition of Eligible Member

A provider usually receives a pre-established amount per member per month—whether or not the member actually receives care. For most populations, the vast majority of members will not receive any mental health care in any given month. However, the provider receiving capitation payments depends on the payments on behalf of the non-patient members. Obviously, the provider has an interest in making sure the health plan accurately tabulates membership—especially when growing membership should increase total capitation payments.

The provider also needs to know whether a particular patient is really a member covered by capitation rather than a fee-for-service patient. Providers need to consider what happens if a patient is assigned to a primary behavioral care physician. The payment for such a patient could resemble a case rate more than a true capitation. To the extent that a provider is not assigned initially, charge-backs might be required to the time of eligibility, which complicates administration.

The capitation rate may vary by a managed care organization's benefit plan or the age and sex of the member. For a Medicaid population, the rate may vary by eligibility category. The total capitation amount the provider actually receives from the health plan may vary from month to month according to these factors and depending on which members the health plan has assigned to the provider. Consequently, the provider has an interest in making sure the health plan keeps accurate details about its members.

Another factor in eligibility determination is the treatment of chronic conditions. The section on "Scope of Services" below addresses some of these issues. Some health plans may limit benefits for individuals with pre-existing conditions. Such limits may reduce the amount of services that the capitated provider will need to provide to patients with pre-existing conditions, thereby reducing the provider's risk. Such limits could also mean that the health plan expects that the provider will not render some medically necessary care to patients with pre-existing conditions.

The health plan also needs to supply a concise definition of what triggers the start of capitation and what triggers the end of capitation. The contract must be clear as to how the health plan assigns members to a psychiatrist. For example, a health plan might assign a psychiatrist to provide care for all members who choose a particular set of primary care physicians (PCPs). The PCPs may act as gatekeepers and refer patients to the psychiatrist.

What Is a Sufficient Volume of Patients?

Many students of college statistics have watched coin flipping experiments that show that the split between Heads and Tails comes closer to 50/50 as the number of coin tosses increases. For a capitation program, the coin-tossing lesson implies the following:

1. Random fluctuations in the number of services will be lower for services that are very frequent.
2. Random fluctuations in costs will be lower for larger capitated populations.

The first item means that the variability in the number of services will be lower for services that occur frequently. For example, for behavioral care, the number of office visits generated by 10,000 people is, on average, greater—and more predictable—than the number of inpatient admissions. Generally, the broader the scope of services and the more predictable the treatment plan, the greater the stability of the costs underlying a capitation rate. In developing a capitation program, providers should analyze the nature of the services and the potential variance in the healthcare system.

The second item also affects the stability of capitation programs. The larger the number of capitated members assigned to a provider, the greater the chance that the provider will see an average spread of risk. Thus, if a capitation program has only 1,000 members, the program has a higher potential for adverse experience than if it has 30,000 members. In the development of a capitation program, the health plan should determine a minimum threshold for the number of members that would make the program viable. A provider should consider actuarial utilization assumptions, expected statistical variance, tolerance for risk, reinsurance arrangements and program structure.

Predictable and Stable Rate
of Claim and Size of Claim

Health plans often calculate a capitation rate as the product of a claim rate (the number of services per 1,000 members) and an average claim size (in dollars per service). If either of these factors is unstable (i.e., high variance), then the likelihood of gains or losses for the provider or the payer increases. Appropriate risk-sharing arrangements could help health plans manage relatively unstable risks. However, both the payer and provider will find it easier to capitate relatively predictable and stable events.

Claim rates and claim sizes for behavioral healthcare programs may not readily meet this criterion. The size of claim may vary substantially from case to case. However, a sound case management approach with clinical pathways can reduce some of the variation on a case to case basis. The frequency of visits and admissions may vary significantly from group to group, and from patient to patient. Benefit limits, while controversial, can also limit the annual or lifetime frequency and size of claims. As with other specialties, new therapies or technologies may increase or decrease the predictability of costs. Ideally, the health plan will structure the capitation program to quickly address changes in the healthcare delivery environment and case management.

Scope of Services

Capitated providers need to understand the health plan's definition of covered services. Hopefully, the payer, provider *and* the member will know the types of included and excluded services. Capitation requires one set of very specific and unambiguous rules. Clear definitions also help streamline contract negotiations between providers and health plans and foster an atmosphere of mutual trust.

The types of services covered can vary considerably. For behavioral health, all parties should know whether the benefits include or exclude pervasive developmental disorders, infantile autism, specific development disorders or organic mental disorders. Defining the scope of services using codes such as CPT-4s, ICD-9s or DRGs can help avoid ambiguity.

Potential Cost Shifting
Across Provider Groups

The flexibility of medical science means that physicians can successfully treat many conditions in a variety of ways. Likewise, for many conditions, general practitioners or a variety of specialists can successfully treat or supervise patients. This flexibility means that the treatment patterns and incentives provided to physicians can have dramatic effects on a provider's cost of treating a capitated population.

For example, some HMOs may encourage primary care physician (PCP) gatekeepers to attempt to treat cases of mild depression, while other plans may, in effect, encourage referrals to psychiatrists. Likewise, the monitoring of patients on drug therapy may fall on either the psychiatrist or the PCP. To the extent the health plan encourages specialists to provide more services—or encourages the PCP to provide fewer services—the specialist needs a higher capitation rate.

Physicians and health plans need to consider the apparent cost-effectiveness of primary care physicians with the potential for increased ultimate costs if effective and decisive specialist treatment is unnecessarily delayed.

Ability to Control Utilization

In order for a provider to control utilization, he or she must have some ability to affect patient flow and patient care. Generally, providers should have a plan to decrease the amount of services provided to capitated patients relative to fee-for-service levels while maintaining the quality of care. The plan may include shifting care to more appropriate settings (along the continuum of behavioral healthcare services) or decreasing the amount of medically unnecessary services.

Under capitation, inappropriate referrals from another provider decrease the chance of financial success. Thus, a capitation program should have incentives to limit inappropriate referrals, whether from health plan administrators or other providers such as primary care physicians. Inappropriate referrals can occur as either too few referrals or too many (services that primary care physicians could provide).

Excessive patient-initiated utilization decreases the chance of success. Thus, if patients perceive the need for certain inappropriate services, the provider may find it difficult to control utilization. This risk may appear as new treatments and technologies emerge. Patients or parent-advocates of children's healthcare may seek the latest therapies, possibly experimental treatments, and these may be expensive, ineffective or redundant. The program design should attempt to control these types of risks, possibly by making the health plan—not the capitated provider—responsible for therapies not explicitly included in the capitation contract.

Fair Negotiations by Both Sides Over Long Term

While the payer ought to compensate providers reasonably, the capitated provider must control costs and not demand increased funds if the provider fails to manage the system. The payer must understand that financial incentives will likely reduce prospective utilization and must be careful not to create payments structures that inappropriately lower capitation rates. If the initial capitation rates prove too high or too low, the payer and provider should accept changes. Also, since many treatments and therapies are evolving and the case management for patients will likely continue evolving, both parties should expect changes to capitation programs.

Often health plans base new programs on sparse data, so both payers and providers should anticipate that results may deviate from those expected. Some new programs have designs that incorporate risk corridors to share among the parties losses or gains from substantial deviations.

Reasonable Links Between Capitated Population and Provider Group

Providers who communicate with the members assigned to them will have a greater chance of success. In particular, communications with non-patient members will help the provider retain membership and capitation income. These communications will also help control administrative problems and enhance patient satisfaction.

Adjusting Capitation Rates

Many health plans use age, sex, family status and geographic factors to adjust capitation rates. Other factors in use (not necessarily actuarially derived) include health status, occupation and industry. Since the capitation rate for an individual is a proxy for an actuarial-based budget of future services, the capitation should vary with expected consumption. For example, ideally, different capitation rates should apply to the Medicaid population based on eligibility category (AFDC, SSI, Foster Care, etc.).

Without factors to adjust capitation rates, the potential for adverse selection increases because capitation rates will, in effect, assume some average cost for all members. This will tend to attract individuals with costs higher than the average implied in the capitation and drive away individuals with lower than average costs. If the health plan uses a classification system that objectively identifies individuals by expected cost, then actuarial factors can appropriately reflect the differing levels of risk.

VI.   RISK MANAGEMENT CHALLENGES FOR SUCCESSFUL CAPITATION PROGRAMS

The main risk management challenges for a successful capitation program include

♦ Inadequate population base
♦ Risk sharing
♦ Catastrophic cases
♦ Actual cost reconciliation
♦ Reserves and margins
♦ Operational issues

Inadequate Population Base

A capitation program may fail unless it has an adequate population base. Groupings of small health plans may create the critical mass necessary for stability. Grouping of geographically disparate providers may also alleviate some of the problems of an inadequate population base, with these providers sharing the gains and losses under capitation.

If grouping cannot resolve the problem, other approaches may work. One alternative is a case-rate that fixes the payment for each patient (or for each type of patient). This approach reduces the need to spread the risk over a population base or over time. The case-rate approach provides an incentive to control consumption of resources for each patient, but does not necessarily reduce the risk that too many members may become patients.

Providers may accept an inadequate population base if anticipated growth meets the minimum expectations within 12 to 18 months. The acceptability of the temporary inadequacy depends on the program's (or provider's) ability to handle adverse deviations from expected costs or expected care. The provider needs to evaluate new or growing programs to determine the financial feasibility of capitation, or if another approach should be used until the population base grows to an adequate size.

Risk Sharing

"Pure" capitation transfers all risk for healthcare services and does not involve risk sharing. (Under pure capitation, the payer still maintains a variety of business and regulatory risks.) However, capitation programs can involve risk sharing or risk corridor adjustments to spread the risk of unexpected or catastrophic cases. The greater the risk sharing, the less the capitation approach transfers risk. Some facility capitation programs involve year-end balance adjustments through risk sharing that can totally eliminate any real risk transfer.

A risk-sharing approach can function as a transition period that allows the provider to become comfortable with assuming greater risk. The provider can analyze whether the pure capitation approach would have resulted in fair compensation. Ideally, risk-sharing approaches need to maintain key capitation incentives. For example, risk-sharing mechanisms should not encourage lax case management through forgiveness of unnecessary medical care.

Catastrophic Cases

Catastrophic cases can adversely impact any capitation approach. Capitated providers often worry about catastrophic cases. The real risk of catastrophic cases varies by capitation approach. There are several ways to alleviate these risks. Two common approaches are individual stop loss and aggregate stop loss. Both of these approaches require converting services rendered into their fee-for-service equivalent costs and comparing these costs to the capitation revenue.

Either health plans or stop loss insurers may provide stop loss coverage. In either case, the stop loss agreement will need to define a method for determining the fee-for-service equivalents of the care rendered.

Individual stop loss compares the fee-for-service equivalent charges for an *individual* patient to a predefined attachment point (e.g., $10,000). The contract usually specifies that these charges accumulate over a calendar year. Once charges have exceeded the attachment point, then the payer or stop loss insurer pays the provider on a fee-for-service basis, either at 100% of the fee-for-service equivalent or at a reduced percent. A reduced percent theoretically encourages continued case management by sharing the cost with the provider. Sometimes stop loss offered by a health plan "forgives" catastrophic claims when evaluating a provider's bonus or incentive payments. If a health plan provides this coverage, the plan may reduce the capitation amount by an actuarially determined amount which reflects the costs of claims above the attachment point. A stop loss insurer will charge a premium for this coverage.

Aggregate stop loss compares the fee-for-service equivalent charges for a group of individuals to a preset aggregate attachment point. Like individual stop loss, the charges are usually accounted for on a calendar-year basis. Aggregate attachment points are often expressed as a percentage above the expected claims or capitation (e.g., 150% of the total capitation payment). Once the fee-for-service equivalents exceed the attachment point, the insurer pays the claims on a fee-for-service basis. The insurer may establish several attachment points with various payment amounts applying. For example, the insurer may pay 50% of the fee-for-service equivalent from 150% to 175% of the capitation payment, and 80% from 175% to 200% of the capitation payment. This approach is more difficult to implement than the individual stop loss approach because the insurer must record and monitor all fee-for-service equivalent amounts.

For either individual or aggregate stop loss, the health plan should set the protection level high enough so that the desired risk transfer still occurs. If all cases fall below the individual stop loss attachment point, then the attachment point has been set too low and no real risk transfer has occurred. For aggregate stop loss, payments should occur rarely over a period of years, otherwise the provider has not assumed an adequate amount of risk.

Actual Cost Reconciliation

Health plans should develop systems to compare actual costs and utilization to capitation program income. However, the provider should not expect that capitation income will equal the fee-for-service equivalent cost. The reconciliation is useful for making appropriate changes to a program to achieve desired results. In performing the actual cost reconciliation, the analyst should use consistent charge levels across all providers in the capitation program. Providers and health plans should develop information systems that will capture sufficient encounter data for the reconciliation.

The actual cost reconciliation can be used to analyze the success of the program and to determine problem areas with the program. The encounter data can be analyzed to determine if the case management protocols have been followed and where further concentration of resources should be directed. The actual cost reconciliation can also be combined with the incentive payment process. Thus, incentive payments can be based on achievement of certain utilization targets measured in the reconciliation.

Reserves and Margins

Reserves and margins can help a provider organization to manage the risk inherent in a capitation contract. Reserves are an essential part of any provider organization that compensates participating providers on a fee-for-service basis. There will be time lags between the time that the service is provided, the time that the service is reported, and the time that the provider is paid. Provider organizations that operate on a pay-as-you-go basis have learned, through hard experience, that by not keeping track of incurred but not reported (IBNR) claims, serious solvency difficulties may result. Provider groups may also desire to maintain contingency reserves for years when medical costs are significantly higher than expected.

IBNR reserves allow a provider organization to perform financial reporting on an accrual basis. If an IBNR liability exists, the provider group should include the liability on its financial statement. The development of the IBNR estimate is based on actuarial techniques that model historical claims payment of the provider system.

Actuaries use a variety of techniques to develop IBNR estimates, but a typical method involves analyzing claim runout patterns. For each month of claims incurred, the actuary estimates the percentage of claims still outstanding. For some healthcare delivery systems, the amount outstanding is fairly stable and predictable over time. For other systems, this factor varies considerably. Factors that affect IBNR liability include, but are not limited to, types of services, claims payment personnel, mail services, catastrophic claims, and out-of-area claims.

Provider groups often maintain contingency reserves to offset unexpectedly high medical or behavioral expenses. The contingency reserve can be set as percentage of expected medical expenses in one year. The contingency reserve can be built up over a few years and replenished if it is partially depleted through adverse medical expenses in one year. The contingency reserve percentage depends on the types of services provided under a capitation contract and the variance associated with those services. Actuaries use claims probability distributions to estimate an optimum contingency reserve based on the provider group's risk tolerance.

Some health plans and providers use withholds to fund budget excesses. In this arrangement, withholds serve as a negative incentive because many providers do not expect to receive a return of the withhold. Under the withhold approach, a portion of each provider payment (fee-for-service or capitation) is deducted to fund a withhold account. If the total medical expenses in one or more budget categories exceeds the expected or budgeted amount, then funds from the withhold account pay for the excesses. This approach provides some protection for adverse claims experience.

Operational Issues

Operations under a capitation arrangement differ significantly from those necessary under a fee-for-service method of reimbursement. Operations for a provider group accepting capitation should resemble traditional insurance company operations. Some operational issues that provider groups should consider when incorporating capitation contracts into their revenue sources include

- Member services
- Provider services
- Management information services

The ability to function effectively under capitation prepayment will rest partially on the effectiveness of these operations. Provider groups need to decide whether they will rent, buy, or develop the personnel and systems to perform these functions.

Member services.   Since providers are paid on a per member per month basis (PMPM) under capitation, the provider must track and manage the member eligibility status. Although some providers rely on health plans, they should also verify eligibility at the point of service. This function can be difficult if the health plan provides limited or untimely data. In addition to the ability to verify eligibility, the provider should also verify the appropriate cost sharing required of the member. The copay amounts are additional revenue for the providers. Capitation rates paid by health plans typically vary inversely with the level of the member cost-sharing requirements.

In addition to providing member verification, provider groups may consider developing customer service departments to provide members with high quality and accurate information. This function will help retain members within the provider group during re-enrollment periods.

Provider services.   Healthcare providers under capitated arrangements often have to work together and coordinate members' healthcare delivery more efficiently than under the fee-for-service compensation system. Provider groups find that they rely on one another to a greater extent than they would have previously expected. Provider groups may consider hiring personnel devoted to maintaining good communication with other providers. Provider groups should also consider hiring personnel with negotiation skills for dealing with compensation of other provider types as well as with the health plans.

Management information systems.   Health plans function not just as financial intermediaries, but as information companies. Insurance companies and health plans devote considerable resources to understand the information generated by their financial intermediary function. This information allows these companies to react relatively quickly to a changing marketplace. Provider groups that accept capitation should also consider the need for sophisticated management information systems. Providers need to determine whether they will rent, buy, or develop the capacity for information processing. Ideally a management information system should at least include the ability to

- Track and analyze encounter specific utilization
- Develop and analyze provider fee schedules
- Profile providers by cost and quality indicators
- Track and analyze members' demographic characteristics
- Track and analyze large claims and reinsurance transactions
- Track and analyze cash flow and financial reporting
- Include on-line referral management
- Include utilization management protocols

VII. ACCESS AND QUALITY ISSUES

We developed the capitation rates in this report by applying actuarial models that apply the relationships among the following factors:

- Benefit limits
- Local costs
- Degree of healthcare management
- Patient cost sharing (deductibles, copays)
- Discounts

While we believe these factors play an important role in determining capitation rates, these factors, by themselves, do not guarantee adequate quality or access. Many physicians have expressed the concern that very low capitation rates simply do not allow the physicians to provide an adequate degree of care. Certainly, poor quality or poor access can occur in plans that appear to provide generous benefits and generous reimbursement. However, the potential for inadequate capitation rates poses a special problem for physicians. If a health plan proposes outrageously low rates, sooner or later providers have to say no. Those types of plans will often generate high levels of complaints by the insured members and may raise serious quality issues.

As mentioned above, the broad demographic characteristics of a given group of individuals can cause mental health utilization to become higher or lower than the costs we have projected here. Certain groups have historically utilized mental health services to a greater or lesser extent than average. Consequently, a capitation payment that would be adequate for an average population could prove inadequate—or overly generous—for a particular group.

Access issues involve the workloads of the physicians, waiting times for appointments and convenience of office hours and treatment sites. These issues vary by region and between rural and urban settings. We encourage physicians to investigate these issues and request specific information from the contracting HMO or other payer.

Degrees of Healthcare Management

The utilization exhibited by different healthcare systems varies widely among programs, even when the programs offer the same benefits and cost sharing. The differences involve how the programs' physicians manage their activity (or on how their activity is managed by the programs). The following table illustrates how aggregate utilization for the commercial population varies by degree of management:

Management Model	Mental Health and Substance Abuse Annual IP Days per 1,000 Members
Loosely Managed Delivery System	110.95
Aggressively Managed Delivery System	17.83

Source.   Milliman & Robertson, Inc.: *Healthcare Management Guidelines, Vol. I: Inpatient and Surgical Care,* 1992.

While the above table illustrates the variability in observed aggregate results, clinicians require protocols that translate these results into actual patient plans. We offer the following principals as an example of the sort of inpatient guidelines that physicians operating in aggressively managed care plans apply:

1. Patients should be treated in the least restrictive setting consistent with quality care. This setting will be closest to best-level functioning. Psychiatric benefits should be provided when psychiatric care coupled with restrictive control is expected to achieve improved mental health status. Less restrictive settings include

    a)   Partial hospital programs
    b)   Residential setting programs
    c)   Day treatment programs

    The hierarchy from acute inpatient, to partial hospital, to a residential setting, to day treatment, to ambulatory care is a hierarchy from most restrictive to least restrictive, from most cost per day to least cost per day, and from most frequent physician services to least frequent physician services. However, short-term crisis intervention in an ambulatory setting may require more frequent, even daily, physician encounters for a short period. The hierarchy of facilities represents options, all of which should be available in managed care plans, from which the most appropriate should be selected for particular patients. The hierarchy does not represent a sequence of care through which all patients need progress.

2. There are few indications for acute inpatient care other than acute short-term controls for the avoidance of danger to self or others, and the initiation and establishment of the structure and content of treatment programs which will continue in less restrictive settings including home and office. Adults and patients with chronic or recurrent problems have the least need for prolonged acute inpatient care.

3. Adolescent patients may require relatively longer acute inpatient stays at their initial presentation with a mental health or psychoactive substance abuse diagnosis of such severity as to require acute inpatient admission. The reasons are

    a)   There may be greater diagnostic uncertainty.
    b)   There may be a greater need for control.
    c)   Family therapy may be a high priority.
    d)   Discharge planning may be more challenging.

e) Acceptance of an appropriate treatment plan may not only provide higher quality, more compliant care, but also avert readmissions.

4. Discharge, disposition and long-term treatment planning should begin at admission and implementation should occur with diagnosis and stability.
5. A semi-weekly review schedule is suggested.
6. Use behavioral home health services to reduce overutilization of emergency room visits and hospital admissions, as a bridge between inpatient and outpatient care, or as ongoing chronic care.

For outpatient mental health services, aggressive management may involve

- Brief and focused therapy approaches
- A "resolve the problem the first time" mentality
- A problem-focused approach to cases
- Timely movement to less restrictive settings without loss of continuity as the patient's condition improves
- Tailoring the treatment within each component to specific patient needs
- Reliance on primary care physicians for prompt diagnosis of physical disorders with behavioral manifestations
- Recognition of potential roles of antecedent medication in psychiatric presentations and removal of potentially offending agents
- Prompt diagnosis of various behavioral disorders and conditions
- Appropriate referrals to behavioral professionals
- Maintenance medication management after stabilization by a psychiatrist
- Coordination of prevention and wellness programs with behavioral and other primary care staff including pain management, elder care, diet, fitness and nutrition

The above principals are based on the Milliman & Robertson, Inc., *Healthcare Management Guidelines.*

In our models, we have used aggressively managed care to mean the consistent application and strict enforcement of these sorts of principals. By contrast, loosely managed care means the sorts of treatment patterns that are typical in non–managed care settings and may have been commonplace in the recent past. They may include some preadmission certification, concurrent review, and hospital audit, but would *not* include inpatient or outpatient care management standards or protocols. Moderately managed care shows the characteristics about halfway between those of aggressively and loosely managed care. Moderate management would include some use of inpatient and outpatient care management standards or protocols with moderate enforcement of such standards.

Because inpatient mental health care costs more than outpatient mental health care, most efforts at utilization management have focused on the inpatient side. More recently, utilization management efforts have begun to affect outpatient care. Consequently, in our scenarios, we have identified the degree of healthcare management for inpatient and outpatient care.

Capitation Rates for the Commercial Population

VIII. CAPITATION RATES FOR THE COMMERCIAL POPULATION

Reported ADM capitation rates for the commercial market vary from about $1 per member per month (PMPM) to over $10 PMPM. Fee-for-service rates, when translated into PMPM units, can be $16 or higher. The age and sex of a particular group and the past claims and diagnosis history of a particular group can push these costs even higher.

Factors That Affect Capitation Rates

Particular groups of individuals with stressful occupations may tend to use ADM benefits more than other groups. For the purposes of this section, we concentrate on a typical population of commercially insured individuals, of the sort that a large insurer or HMO may present to a ADM provider. That is, we do not consider the age or sex characteristics of the population or the past claims experience. Providers who may have to deal with specialized populations or employer groups should have their advisors consider these other factors.

Many different factors can affect ADM costs, but those that can have a major impact are far fewer. The following characteristics do have major effects on ADM benefit utilization of typical commercial populations:

- *The extent of benefits.* Plans that offer unlimited coverage for inpatient days and outpatients visits can cost about twice as much as plans with very limited coverage, all other things equal.
- *The local area's costs.* Low-cost areas in the U.S. have costs that are half as much as the costs in high-cost areas, all other things equal.
- *Copay levels.* Plans that require no inpatient copay and a $10 outpatient copay have costs that are 25% greater than plans that require a $500 inpatient copay and $40 per outpatient visit, all other things equal.
- *Type of healthcare management.* Plans that aggressively manage inpatient and outpatient care can have costs that are about 50% lower than unmanaged plans, all other things equal.
- *Discount level.* Plans that, in effect, pay a large discount compared to fee-for-service levels can reduce costs considerably compared to those that offer a lower discount. While most capitation arrangements imply some discount, these can range from under 20% to over 50%.

The following chart summarizes the estimated magnitude of *potential* cost impact that individual factors can have on costs. Please note that these effects may not be cumulative across factors due to the interactive effects of low plan benefits, utilization management, local cost levels, etc.

Factor	Potential Cost Reductions (Approximate) From National Average Fee-for-Service Levels
Extent of Benefits	50%
Local Area Cost	30%
Copays	25%
Type of Management	50%
Discount Level	50%

In our report we show estimated capitation rates for the following variations:

Extent of benefits per calendar year (plan type)—4 variations

♦ Unlimited inpatient days and outpatient visits (parity with medical/surgical benefits)
♦ 45 inpatient days and 30 outpatient visits
♦ 30 inpatient days and 20 outpatient visits
♦ 15 inpatient days and 45 outpatient visits

Local area cost—3 variations

♦ National average (undiscounted costs of about $958 per IP day, $117 per IP visit, $123 per OP visit)
♦ National average + 20% (unit price plus utilization)
♦ National average – 20% (unit price plus utilization)

Copays—2 variations

♦ $0 per inpatient admission, $10 per professional visit
♦ $200 per inpatient admission, $25 per professional visit

Type of healthcare management—5 variations

♦ Unmanaged
♦ Moderately managed—inpatient only
♦ Moderately managed—inpatient and outpatient
♦ Aggressively managed—inpatient only
♦ Aggressively managed—inpatient and outpatient

Discount level—3 levels

♦ 20% discount
♦ 30% discount
♦ 40% discount

We present utilization and cost per service rates for a selection of our benefit plan variations and the capitation rates for the 360 combinations (4 x 3 x 2 x 5 x 3) of these variations in the following tables.

Certain combinations of these factors (e.g., low benefit plans combined with low local cost levels, aggressive care management, high patient cost sharing, and large provider discounts) produce low capitation rates. We recognize that the APA is very concerned that low capitation rates simply may not allow physicians to provide an adequate amount of care. Certainly, poor quality or poor access can occur in plans that appear to offer generous benefits or reimbursement. We do not intend for this report to be used by organizations to justify inadequate capitation rates for ADM providers. Rather, we present rates associated with these various combinations of factors in order to provide general guidance and education to APA members on these capitation issues.

No explicit margins or allowances for administrative expenses, coordination of benefits, stop loss reinsurance, adverse risks, or margins for profits and/or contingencies beyond those implicitly provided within the average costs per unit of service have been used.

Commercial Population Utilization

Assumes National Average Area w/ 30% Discount,
Copays of $200 per Admit & $25 per OP Visit
Annual Rates per 1,000 Members

Benefits / Management Type	15 IP Days, 15 IP Visits, 45 OP Visits			30 IP Days, 30 IP Visits, 20 OP Visits			45 IP Days, 45 IP Visits, 30 OP Visits			Unlimited IP Days, IP Visits, OP Visits		
	IP Days	IP Visits	OP Visits	IP Days	IP Visits	OP Visits	IP Days	IP Visits	OP Visits	IP Days	IP Visits	OP Visits
Aggressively Managed - I/P & O/P	18	26	369	18	26	334	18	26	334	23	34	392
Aggressively Managed - I/P Only	18	26	737	18	26	576	18	26	668	23	34	783
Moderately Managed - I/P & O/P	36	47	442	50	65	346	54	70	401	70	91	470
Moderately Managed - I/P Only	36	47	614	50	65	480	54	70	557	70	91	653
Loosely Managed (Unmanaged)	66	75	491	91	104	384	98	112	445	128	145	522

Commercial Population Cost per Service
Assumes Moderately Managed - I/P & O/P Plan of 30 IP Days, 30 IP Visits, 20 OP Visits
With Copays of $200 per Admit & $25 per OP Visit

	40 % Discount			30 % Discount			20 % Discount		
	IP Days	IP Visits	OP Visits	IP Days	IP Visits	OP Visits	IP Days	IP Visits	OP Visits
National Average + 20 %	$766.71	$82.67	$80.65	$894.49	$96.44	$94.09	$1,022.28	$110.22	$107.53
National Average	621.10	75.61	73.76	724.61	88.21	86.06	828.13	100.81	98.35
National Average - 20 %	531.78	69.42	67.72	620.40	80.99	79.01	709.03	92.55	90.30

Commercial Population Capitation Rates
Benefit Plan : 15 IP Days, 15 IP Visits, 45 OP Visits
Copays : $0 per Admit, $10 per OP Visit

Care Management	Cost Level	Discount Level	PMPM Rate
Loosely Managed (Unmanaged)	National Avg. + 20%	40%	*8.03
		30%	9.45
		20%	11.02
	National Avg.	40%	6.47
		30%	7.62
		20%	8.88
	National Avg. - 20%	40%	5.14
		30%	6.06
		20%	6.99
Moderately Managed - I/P Only	National Avg. + 20%	40%	7.12
		30%	8.42
		20%	9.90
	National Avg.	40%	5.78
		30%	6.83
		20%	8.03
	National Avg. - 20%	40%	4.62
		30%	5.47
		20%	6.33
Moderately Managed - I/P & O/P	National Avg. + 20%	40%	5.89
		30%	6.95
		20%	8.13
	National Avg.	40%	4.76
		30%	5.62
		20%	6.59
	National Avg. - 20%	40%	3.81
		30%	4.50
		20%	5.20
Aggressively Managed - I/P Only	National Avg. + 20%	40%	6.68
		30%	7.92
		20%	9.39
	National Avg.	40%	5.46
		30%	6.47
		20%	7.69
	National Avg. - 20%	40%	4.49
		30%	5.35
		20%	6.18
Aggressively Managed - I/P & O/P	National Avg. + 20%	40%	4.02
		30%	4.76
		20%	5.61
	National Avg.	40%	3.30
		30%	3.90
		20%	4.60
	National Avg. - 20%	40%	2.74
		30%	3.25
		20%	3.75

No explicit margins or allowances for administrative expenses, coordination of benefits, stop loss reinsurance, adverse risks, or margins for profits and/or contingencies beyond those implicitly provided within the average costs per unit of service have been used.

Commercial Population Capitation Rates
Benefit Plan : 15 IP Days, 15 IP Visits, 45 OP Visits
Copays : $200 per Admit, $25 per OP Visit

Care Management	Cost Level	Discount Level	PMPM Rate
Loosely Managed (Unmanaged)	National Avg. + 20%	40%	6.81
		30%	8.24
		20%	9.74
	National Avg.	40%	5.40
		30%	6.56
		20%	7.76
	National Avg. - 20%	40%	4.16
		30%	5.08
		20%	6.04
Moderately Managed - I/P Only	National Avg. + 20%	40%	5.67
		30%	7.00
		20%	8.36
	National Avg.	40%	4.50
		30%	5.58
		20%	6.69
	National Avg. - 20%	40%	3.46
		30%	4.30
		20%	5.19
Moderately Managed - I/P & O/P	National Avg. + 20%	40%	4.81
		30%	5.91
		20%	7.01
	National Avg.	40%	3.83
		30%	4.70
		20%	5.60
	National Avg. - 20%	40%	2.94
		30%	3.63
		20%	4.35
Aggressively Managed - I/P Only	National Avg. + 20%	40%	4.98
		30%	6.26
		20%	7.60
	National Avg.	40%	3.99
		30%	5.02
		20%	6.12
	National Avg. - 20%	40%	3.12
		30%	3.97
		20%	4.85
Aggressively Managed - I/P & O/P	National Avg. + 20%	40%	3.15
		30%	3.90
		20%	4.69
	National Avg.	40%	2.54
		30%	3.14
		20%	3.80
	National Avg. - 20%	40%	2.11
		30%	2.60
		20%	3.06

No explicit margins or allowances for administrative expenses, coordination of benefits, stop loss reinsurance, adverse risks, or margins for profits and/or contingencies beyond those implicitly provided within the average costs per unit of service have been used.

Commercial Population Capitation Rates
Benefit Plan : 30 IP Days, 30 IP Visits, 20 OP Visits
Copays : $0 per Admit, $10 per OP Visit

Care Management	Cost Level	Discount Level	PMPM Rate
Loosely Managed (Unmanaged)	National Avg. + 20%	40%	8.98
		30%	10.54
		20%	12.23
	National Avg.	40%	7.21
		30%	8.47
		20%	9.84
	National Avg. - 20%	40%	5.71
		30%	6.72
		20%	7.72
Moderately Managed - I/P Only	National Avg. + 20%	40%	7.21
		30%	8.48
		20%	9.92
	National Avg.	40%	5.82
		30%	6.86
		20%	8.02
	National Avg. - 20%	40%	4.63
		30%	5.47
		20%	6.31
Moderately Managed - I/P & O/P	National Avg. + 20%	40%	6.24
		30%	7.34
		20%	8.54
	National Avg.	40%	5.02
		30%	5.91
		20%	6.89
	National Avg. - 20%	40%	3.99
		30%	4.70
		20%	5.41
Aggressively Managed - I/P Only	National Avg. + 20%	40%	5.52
		30%	6.54
		20%	7.73
	National Avg.	40%	4.52
		30%	5.35
		20%	6.33
	National Avg. - 20%	40%	3.72
		30%	4.42
		20%	5.11
Aggressively Managed - I/P & O/P	National Avg. + 20%	40%	3.45
		30%	4.07
		20%	4.79
	National Avg.	40%	2.91
		30%	3.44
		20%	3.97
	National Avg. - 20%	40%	2.58
		30%	3.07
		20%	3.53

No explicit margins or allowances for administrative expenses, coordination of benefits, stop loss reinsurance, adverse risks, or margins for profits and/or contingencies beyond those implicitly provided within the average costs per unit of service have been used.

Commercial Population Capitation Rates
Benefit Plan : 30 IP Days, 30 IP Visits, 20 OP Visits
Copays : $200 per Admit, $25 per OP Visit

Care Management	Cost Level	Discount Level	PMPM Rate
Loosely Managed (Unmanaged)	National Avg. + 20%	40%	7.99
		30%	9.58
		20%	11.20
	National Avg.	40%	6.35
		30%	7.61
		20%	8.93
	National Avg. - 20%	40%	4.96
		30%	5.94
		20%	6.95
Moderately Managed - I/P Only	National Avg. + 20%	40%	6.05
		30%	7.35
		20%	8.69
	National Avg.	40%	4.80
		30%	5.86
		20%	6.96
	National Avg. - 20%	40%	3.70
		30%	4.54
		20%	5.40
Moderately Managed - I/P & O/P	National Avg. + 20%	40%	5.39
		30%	6.49
		20%	7.63
	National Avg.	40%	4.27
		30%	5.18
		20%	6.11
	National Avg. - 20%	40%	3.46
		30%	4.17
		20%	4.87
Aggressively Managed - I/P Only	National Avg. + 20%	40%	4.18
		30%	5.23
		20%	6.32
	National Avg.	40%	3.35
		30%	4.20
		20%	5.10
	National Avg. - 20%	40%	2.64
		30%	3.34
		20%	4.06
Aggressively Managed - I/P & O/P	National Avg. + 20%	40%	2.86
		30%	3.47
		20%	4.07
	National Avg.	40%	2.44
		30%	2.97
		20%	3.50
	National Avg. - 20%	40%	2.11
		30%	2.60
		20%	3.06

No explicit margins or allowances for administrative expenses, coordination of benefits, stop loss reinsurance, adverse risks, or margins for profits and/or contingencies beyond those implicitly provided within the average costs per unit of service have been used.

Commercial Population Capitation Rates
Benefit Plan : 45 IP Days, 45 IP Visits, 30 OP Visits
Copays : $0 per Admit, $10 per OP Visit

Care Management	Cost Level	Discount Level	PMPM Rate
Loosely Managed (Unmanaged)	National Avg. + 20%	40%	9.90
		30%	11.63
		20%	13.50
	National Avg.	40%	7.96
		30%	9.35
		20%	10.86
	National Avg. - 20%	40%	6.30
		30%	7.41
		20%	8.53
Moderately Managed - I/P Only	National Avg. + 20%	40%	8.05
		30%	9.48
		20%	11.09
	National Avg.	40%	6.50
		30%	7.66
		20%	8.97
	National Avg. - 20%	40%	5.18
		30%	6.13
		20%	7.07
Moderately Managed - I/P & O/P	National Avg. + 20%	40%	6.93
		30%	8.15
		20%	9.49
	National Avg.	40%	5.58
		30%	6.56
		20%	7.67
	National Avg. - 20%	40%	4.44
		30%	5.24
		20%	6.04
Aggressively Managed - I/P Only	National Avg. + 20%	40%	6.20
		30%	7.35
		20%	8.70
	National Avg.	40%	5.06
		30%	6.01
		20%	7.11
	National Avg. - 20%	40%	4.16
		30%	4.95
		20%	5.73
Aggressively Managed - I/P & O/P	National Avg. + 20%	40%	3.80
		30%	4.48
		20%	5.28
	National Avg.	40%	3.10
		30%	3.66
		20%	4.31
	National Avg. - 20%	40%	2.58
		30%	3.07
		20%	3.53

No explicit margins or allowances for administrative expenses, coordination of benefits, stop loss reinsurance, adverse risks, or margins for profits and/or contingencies beyond those implicitly provided within the average costs per unit of service have been used.

Commercial Population Capitation Rates
Benefit Plan : 45 IP Days, 45 IP Visits, 30 OP Visits
Copays : $200 per Admit, $25 per OP Visit

Care Management	Cost Level	Discount Level	PMPM Rate
Loosely Managed (Unmanaged)	National Avg. + 20%	40%	8.78
		30%	10.53
		20%	12.33
	National Avg.	40%	6.97
		30%	8.38
		20%	9.83
	National Avg. - 20%	40%	5.40
		30%	6.52
		20%	7.66
Moderately Managed - I/P Only	National Avg. + 20%	40%	6.73
		30%	8.18
		20%	9.69
	National Avg.	40%	5.33
		30%	6.51
		20%	7.75
	National Avg. - 20%	40%	4.11
		30%	5.07
		20%	6.03
Moderately Managed - I/P & O/P	National Avg. + 20%	40%	5.95
		30%	7.19
		20%	8.46
	National Avg.	40%	4.72
		30%	5.71
		20%	6.77
	National Avg. - 20%	40%	3.65
		30%	4.46
		20%	5.27
Aggressively Managed - I/P Only	National Avg. + 20%	40%	4.66
		30%	5.84
		20%	7.07
	National Avg.	40%	3.71
		30%	4.68
		20%	5.68
	National Avg. - 20%	40%	2.92
		30%	3.70
		20%	4.51
Aggressively Managed - I/P & O/P	National Avg. + 20%	40%	2.99
		30%	3.70
		20%	4.43
	National Avg.	40%	2.44
		30%	2.98
		20%	3.57
	National Avg. - 20%	40%	2.11
		30%	2.60
		20%	3.06

No explicit margins or allowances for administrative expenses, coordination of benefits, stop loss reinsurance, adverse risks, or margins for profits and/or contingencies beyond those implicitly provided within the average costs per unit of service have been used.

Commercial Population Capitation Rates
Benefit Plan : Unlimited IP Days, IP Visits, OP Visits
Copays : $0 per Admit, $10 per OP Visit

Care Management	Cost Level	Discount Level	PMPM Rate
Loosely Managed (Unmanaged)	National Avg. + 20%	40%	12.49
		30%	14.66
		20%	16.99
	National Avg.	40%	10.03
		30%	11.78
		20%	13.66
	National Avg. - 20%	40%	7.95
		30%	9.34
		20%	10.74
Moderately Managed - I/P Only	National Avg. + 20%	40%	9.97
		30%	11.74
		20%	13.71
	National Avg.	40%	8.05
		30%	9.48
		20%	11.09
	National Avg. - 20%	40%	6.41
		30%	7.56
		20%	8.72
Moderately Managed - I/P & O/P	National Avg. + 20%	40%	8.65
		30%	10.18
		20%	11.84
	National Avg.	40%	6.98
		30%	8.20
		20%	9.55
	National Avg. - 20%	40%	5.54
		30%	6.52
		20%	7.51
Aggressively Managed - I/P Only	National Avg. + 20%	40%	7.46
		30%	8.83
		20%	10.46
	National Avg.	40%	6.04
		30%	7.18
		20%	8.51
	National Avg. - 20%	40%	4.87
		30%	5.79
		20%	6.70
Aggressively Managed - I/P & O/P	National Avg. + 20%	40%	4.64
		30%	5.48
		20%	6.44
	National Avg.	40%	3.75
		30%	4.44
		20%	5.22
	National Avg. - 20%	40%	3.01
		30%	3.56
		20%	4.12

No explicit margins or allowances for administrative expenses, coordination of benefits, stop loss reinsurance, adverse risks, or margins for profits and/or contingencies beyond those implicitly provided within the average costs per unit of service have been used.

Commercial Population Capitation Rates
Benefit Plan : Unlimited IP Days, IP Visits, OP Visits
Copays : $200 per Admit, $25 per OP Visit

Care Management	Cost Level	Discount Level	PMPM Rate
Loosely Managed (Unmanaged)	National Avg. + 20%	40%	11.21
		30%	13.39
		20%	15.64
	National Avg.	40%	8.90
		30%	10.66
		20%	12.47
	National Avg. - 20%	40%	6.91
		30%	8.31
		20%	9.73
Moderately Managed - I/P Only	National Avg. + 20%	40%	8.43
		30%	10.24
		20%	12.09
	National Avg.	40%	6.70
		30%	8.15
		20%	9.66
	National Avg. - 20%	40%	5.17
		30%	6.32
		20%	7.52
Moderately Managed - I/P & O/P	National Avg. + 20%	40%	7.52
		30%	9.07
		20%	10.65
	National Avg.	40%	5.98
		30%	7.22
		20%	8.51
	National Avg. - 20%	40%	4.63
		30%	5.61
		20%	6.62
Aggressively Managed - I/P Only	National Avg. + 20%	40%	5.66
		30%	7.07
		20%	8.55
	National Avg.	40%	4.47
		30%	5.64
		20%	6.84
	National Avg. - 20%	40%	3.42
		30%	4.34
		20%	5.30
Aggressively Managed - I/P & O/P	National Avg. + 20%	40%	3.72
		30%	4.58
		20%	5.46
	National Avg.	40%	2.93
		30%	3.64
		20%	4.37
	National Avg. - 20%	40%	2.27
		30%	2.80
		20%	3.38

No explicit margins or allowances for administrative expenses, coordination of benefits, stop loss reinsurance, adverse risks, or margins for profits and/or contingencies beyond those implicitly provided within the average costs per unit of service have been used.

Capitation Rates for the Medicare Population

IX.   Capitation Rates for the Medicare Population

Since the Health Care Financing Administration (HCFA) published final regulations to allow eligible organizations to provide care for Medicare enrollees on a risk basis, more than 150 organizations have obtained approval for such risk contracts. Many of these organizations have found that they have numerous problems in controlling costs under a risk contract. Others have contracted successfully. Many more organizations have evaluated Medicare risk contracting for their organizations and decided against pursuing it.

Medicare risk contractors are exposed to a number of risks, including

> **Retention risk**   The risk that expenses to the organization (cost of providing care plus retention) will exceed revenues (Medicare APACE payments plus supplemental premium payments).
>
> **Trend risk**   The risk that trends associated with medical and behavioral care costs will outpace the trend assumption used in APACE calculations.
>
> **Political risk**   The risk that the APACE will be inappropriately low because of politically motivated Medicare savings estimates that HCFA may incorporate in APACE calculations.
>
> **COB risk**   The risk that organizations will not recover the coordination of benefits amounts implicitly assumed in the APACE calculations for Medicare secondary payer and other COB items.
>
> **Out-of-plan risk**   The risk that Medicare enrollees will overutilize out-of-plan care (both emergency and urgently needed care) for which the organization is financially responsible.
>
> **Competition risk**   The risk that other organizations will enter the Medicare risk process with inadequate premiums and unrealistic expectations.

It is within this context that behavioral healthcare providers may be capitated to provide behavioral healthcare services to Medicare risk contract enrollees.

There are several factors applicable to the Medicare population that can contribute to cost variations in the provision of behavioral healthcare services, including

- Differences in utilization levels of inpatient vs. outpatient services, prior to utilization management application
- Degree of utilization management (managed care efficiency) both for inpatient and outpatient services
- Variations in the Medicare allowable charges per unit for professional services

- Variations in hospital and facility charges per day
- Variations in benefit plan designs concerning insured copayments
- Variations by state in psychologist hospital privileges

We have incorporated these variables within our Medicare behavioral cost estimates by using the following:

- Three different utilization scenarios prior to the application of managed care efficiencies (Mid-level or National, High, and Low)
- Three different prevailing average cost levels for inpatient and Medicare-allowed outpatient services
- Five different managed care scenarios, representing unmanaged, moderately managed inpatient care with unmanaged outpatient care, moderately managed inpatient and outpatient care, aggressively managed inpatient care with unmanaged outpatient care, and aggressively managed delivery of inpatient care and outpatient care services
- Two different scenarios for the effective discount to prevailing cost levels
- Three different plan designs reflecting various insured copayments

Certain combinations of these factors (e.g., low benefit plans combined with low local cost levels, aggressive care management, high patient cost sharing, and large provider discounts) produce low capitation rates. We recognize that the APA is very concerned that low capitation rates simply may not allow physicians to provide an adequate amount of care. Certainly, poor quality or poor access can occur in plans that appear to offer generous benefits or reimbursement. We do not intend for this report to be used by organizations to justify inadequate capitation rates for ADM providers. Rather, we present rates associated with these various combinations of factors in order to provide general guidance and education to APA members on these capitation issues.

No explicit margins or allowances for administrative expenses, coordination of benefits, stop loss reinsurance, or margins for profits and/or contingencies beyond those implicitly provided within the average charges per unit of service have been used.

The following tables present our Medicare scenario assumptions and the corresponding behavioral cost estimates for these scenarios.

MEDICARE UTILIZATION ASSUMPTIONS
MID-LEVEL (NATIONAL)

Managed Care Scenario	Inpatient Days (Annual Per 1,000)	Inpatient Visits (Annual Per 1,000)	Outpatient Visits (Annual Per 1,000)
(1) Unmanaged	50	55	385
(2)Moderately Managed I/P Only	33	41	420
(3)Moderately Managed I/P & O/P	33	41	300
(4)Aggressively Managed I/P Only	19	28	447
(5)Aggressively Managed I/P & O/P	19	28	223

MEDICARE UTILIZATION ASSUMPTIONS- HIGH LEVEL

Managed Care Scenario	Inpatient Days (Annual Per 1,000)	Inpatient Visits (Annual Per 1,000)	Outpatient Visits (Annual Per 1,000)
(1)Unmanaged	65	72	525
(2)Moderately Managed I/P Only	43	54	572
(3)Moderately Managed I/P & O/P	43	54	410
(4)Aggressively Managed I/P Only	25	36	609
(5)Aggressively Managed I/P & O/P	25	36	305

MEDICARE UTILIZATION ASSUMPTIONS - LOW LEVEL

Managed Care Scenario	Inpatient Days (Annual Per 1,000)	Inpatient Visits (Annual Per 1,000)	Outpatient Visits (Annual Per 1,000)
(1)Unmanaged	35	39	275
(2)Moderately Managed I/P Only	26	32	295
(3)Moderately Managed I/P & O/P	26	32	245
(4)Aggressively Managed I/P Only	19	28	310
(5)Aggressively Managed I/P & O/P	19	28	223

PREVAILING AVERAGE COSTS

Scenario	I/P per Day	Professional I/P (Per Visit)	Professional O/P (Per Visit)
High	$1,000	$85	$80
Mid	$ 850	$80	$75
Low	$ 700	$75	$70

EFFECTIVE DISCOUNTS

Scenario	Percent of Medicare Allowable
No Discount	100%
10% Discount	90%
20% Discount	80%

PLAN DESIGNS

Plan	Inpatient Copay	Professional Copay
1)	$0 per admit	$0 per visit
2)	$250 per admit	$5 per visit
3)	$500 per admit	$10 per visit

Medicare Population Capitation Rates
Unmanaged Care
Copayments: None

Utilization Level	Cost Level	% of Medicare Allowable	PMPM Rate
National	National	100%	$6.31
		90%	$5.68
		80%	$5.05
	High	100%	$7.12
		90%	$6.41
		80%	$5.70
	Low	100%	$5.51
		90%	$4.96
		80%	$4.41
High	National	100%	$8.37
		90%	$7.53
		80%	$6.69
	High	100%	$9.43
		90%	$8.48
		80%	$7.54
	Low	100%	$7.30
		90%	$6.57
		80%	$5.84
Low	National	100%	$4.46
		90%	$4.01
		80%	$3.57
	High	100%	$5.03
		90%	$4.52
		80%	$4.02
	Low	100%	$3.89
		90%	$3.50
		80%	$3.11

LEGEND

	Utilization Levels		
	National	High	Low
Annual Inpatient Days/1000	50	65	35
Annual Inpatient Visits/1000	55	72	39
AnnualOutpatient Visits/1000	385	525	275
	Cost Levels		
	National	High	Low
Cost per Inpatient Day	$850	$1,000	$700
Cost per Inpatient Visit	$80	$85	$75
Cost per Outpatient Visit	$75	$80	$70

No explicit margins or allowances for administrative expenses, coordination of benefits, stop loss reinsurance, adverse risks, or margins for profits and/or contingencies beyond those implicitly provided within the average costs per unit of service have been used.

Medicare Population Capitation Rates
Unmanaged Care
Copayments: $250 per I/P Admit, $5 per Visit

Utilization Level	Cost Level	% of Medicare Allowable	PMPM Rate
National	National	100%	$6.03
		90%	$5.43
		80%	$4.82
	High	100%	$6.84
		90%	$6.15
		80%	$5.47
	Low	100%	$5.22
		90%	$4.70
		80%	$4.18
High	National	100%	$8.01
		90%	$7.21
		80%	$6.41
	High	100%	$9.07
		90%	$8.16
		80%	$7.25
	Low	100%	$6.95
		90%	$6.25
		80%	$5.56
Low	National	100%	$4.25
		90%	$3.82
		80%	$3.40
	High	100%	$4.82
		90%	$4.33
		80%	$3.85
	Low	100%	$3.68
		90%	$3.31
		80%	$2.94

LEGEND

	Utilization Levels		
	National	High	Low
Annual Inpatient Days/1000	50	65	35
Annual Inpatient Visits/1000	55	72	39
AnnualOutpatient Visits/1000	385	525	275

	Cost Levels		
	National	High	Low
Cost per Inpatient Day	$850	$1,000	$700
Cost per Inpatient Visit	$80	$85	$75
Cost per Outpatient Visit	$75	$80	$70

No explicit margins or allowances for administrative expenses, coordination of benefits, stop loss reinsurance, adverse risks, or margins for profits and/or contingencies beyond those implicitly provided within the average costs per unit of service have been used.

Medicare Population Capitation Rates
Unmanaged Care
Copayments: $500 per I/P Admit, $10 per Visit

Utilization Level	Cost Level	% of Medicare Allowable	PMPM Rate
National	National	100%	$5.75
		90%	$5.17
		80%	$4.60
	High	100%	$6.55
		90%	$5.90
		80%	$5.24
	Low	100%	$4.94
		90%	$4.44
		80%	$3.95
High	National	100%	$7.65
		90%	$6.88
		80%	$6.12
	High	100%	$8.71
		90%	$7.84
		80%	$6.97
	Low	100%	$6.59
		90%	$5.93
		80%	$5.27
Low	National	100%	$4.04
		90%	$3.63
		80%	$3.23
	High	100%	$4.61
		90%	$4.15
		80%	$3.69
	Low	100%	$3.47
		90%	$3.12
		80%	$2.78

LEGEND

Utilization Levels	National	High	Low
Annual Inpatient Days/1000	50	65	35
Annual Inpatient Visits/1000	55	72	39
AnnualOutpatient Visits/1000	385	525	275

Cost Levels	National	High	Low
Cost per Inpatient Day	$850	$1,000	$700
Cost per Inpatient Visit	$80	$85	$75
Cost per Outpatient Visit	$75	$80	$70

No explicit margins or allowances for administrative expenses, coordination of benefits, stop loss reinsurance, adverse risks, or margins for profits and/or contingencies beyond those implicitly provided within the average costs per unit of service have been used.

Medicare Population Capitation Rates
Moderately Managed Care, Inpatient Only
Copayments: None

Utilization Level	Cost Level	% of Medicare Allowable	PMPM Rate
National	National	100%	$5.24
		90%	$4.71
		80%	$4.19
	High	100%	$5.84
		90%	$5.26
		80%	$4.67
	Low	100%	$4.63
		90%	$4.17
		80%	$3.71
High	National	100%	$6.98
		90%	$6.28
		80%	$5.58
	High	100%	$7.78
		90%	$7.00
		80%	$6.22
	Low	100%	$6.18
		90%	$5.56
		80%	$4.95
Low	National	100%	$3.90
		90%	$3.51
		80%	$3.12
	High	100%	$4.36
		90%	$3.92
		80%	$3.49
	Low	100%	$3.44
		90%	$3.09
		80%	$2.75

LEGEND

	Utilization Levels		
	National	High	Low
Annual Inpatient Days/1000	33	43	26
Annual Inpatient Visits/1000	41	54	32
AnnualOutpatient Visits/1000	420	572	295

	Cost Levels		
	National	High	Low
Cost per Inpatient Day	$850	$1,000	$700
Cost per Inpatient Visit	$80	$85	$75
Cost per Outpatient Visit	$75	$80	$70

No explicit margins or allowances for administrative expenses, coordination of benefits, stop loss reinsurance, adverse risks, or margins for profits and/or contingencies beyond those implicitly provided within the average costs per unit of service have been used.

Medicare Population Capitation Rates
Moderately Managed Care, Inpatient Only
Copayments: $250 per I/P Admit, $5 per Visit

Utilization Level	Cost Level	% of Medicare Allowable	PMPM Rate
National	National	100%	$4.97
		90%	$4.47
		80%	$3.98
	High	100%	$5.58
		90%	$5.02
		80%	$4.46
	Low	100%	$4.37
		90%	$3.93
		80%	$3.49
High	National	100%	$6.64
		90%	$5.98
		80%	$5.31
	High	100%	$7.44
		90%	$6.70
		80%	$5.95
	Low	100%	$5.84
		90%	$5.26
		80%	$4.67
Low	National	100%	$3.70
		90%	$3.33
		80%	$2.96
	High	100%	$4.16
		90%	$3.75
		80%	$3.33
	Low	100%	$3.24
		90%	$2.92
		80%	$2.59

LEGEND

	Utilization Levels		
	National	High	Low
Annual Inpatient Days/1000	33	43	26
Annual Inpatient Visits/1000	41	54	32
AnnualOutpatient Visits/1000	420	572	295
	Cost Levels		
	National	High	Low
Cost per Inpatient Day	$850	$1,000	$700
Cost per Inpatient Visit	$80	$85	$75
Cost per Outpatient Visit	$75	$80	$70

No explicit margins or allowances for administrative expenses, coordination of benefits, stop loss reinsurance, adverse risks, or margins for profits and/or contingencies beyond those implicitly provided within the average costs per unit of service have been used.

Medicare Population Capitation Rates
Moderately Managed Care, Inpatient Only
Copayments: $500 per I/P Admit, $10 per Visit

Utilization Level	Cost Level	% of Medicare Allowable	PMPM Rate
National	National	100%	$4.71
		90%	$4.24
		80%	$3.77
	High	100%	$5.31
		90%	$4.78
		80%	$4.25
	Low	100%	$4.10
		90%	$3.69
		80%	$3.28
High	National	100%	$6.30
		90%	$5.67
		80%	$5.04
	High	100%	$7.10
		90%	$6.39
		80%	$5.68
	Low	100%	$5.50
		90%	$4.95
		80%	$4.40
Low	National	100%	$3.51
		90%	$3.15
		80%	$2.80
	High	100%	$3.97
		90%	$3.57
		80%	$3.17
	Low	100%	$3.04
		90%	$2.74
		80%	$2.44

LEGEND

Utilization Levels	National	High	Low
Annual Inpatient Days/1000	33	43	26
Annual Inpatient Visits/1000	41	54	32
AnnualOutpatient Visits/1000	420	572	295

Cost Levels	National	High	Low
Cost per Inpatient Day	$850	$1,000	$700
Cost per Inpatient Visit	$80	$85	$75
Cost per Outpatient Visit	$75	$80	$70

No explicit margins or allowances for administrative expenses, coordination of benefits, stop loss reinsurance, adverse risks, or margins for profits and/or contingencies beyond those implicitly provided within the average costs per unit of service have been used.

Medicare Population Capitation Rates
Moderately Managed Care, Inpatient and Outpatient
Copayments: None

Utilization Level	Cost Level	% of Medicare Allowable	PMPM Rate
National	National	100%	$4.49
		90%	$4.04
		80%	$3.59
	High	100%	$5.04
		90%	$4.54
		80%	$4.03
	Low	100%	$3.93
		90%	$3.54
		80%	$3.15
High	National	100%	$5.97
		90%	$5.37
		80%	$4.77
	High	100%	$6.70
		90%	$6.03
		80%	$5.36
	Low	100%	$5.24
		90%	$4.71
		80%	$4.19
Low	National	100%	$3.59
		90%	$3.23
		80%	$2.87
	High	100%	$4.03
		90%	$3.62
		80%	$3.22
	Low	100%	$3.15
		90%	$2.83
		80%	$2.52

LEGEND

Utilization Levels	National	High	Low
Annual Inpatient Days/1000	33	43	26
Annual Inpatient Visits/1000	41	54	32
AnnualOutpatient Visits/1000	300	410	245

Cost Levels	National	High	Low
Cost per Inpatient Day	$850	$1,000	$700
Cost per Inpatient Visit	$80	$85	$75
Cost per Outpatient Visit	$75	$80	$70

No explicit margins or allowances for administrative expenses, coordination of benefits, stop loss reinsurance, adverse risks, or margins for profits and/or contingencies beyond those implicitly provided within the average costs per unit of service have been used.

Medicare Population Capitation Rates
Moderately Managed Care, Inpatient and Outpatient
Copayments: $250 per I/P Admit, $5 per Visit

Utilization Level	Cost Level	% of Medicare Allowable	PMPM Rate
National	National	100%	$4.27
		90%	$3.84
		80%	$3.42
	High	100%	$4.83
		90%	$4.34
		80%	$3.86
	Low	100%	$3.72
		90%	$3.35
		80%	$2.97
High	National	100%	$5.70
		90%	$5.13
		80%	$4.56
	High	100%	$6.43
		90%	$5.78
		80%	$5.14
	Low	100%	$4.97
		90%	$4.47
		80%	$3.97
Low	National	100%	$3.41
		90%	$3.07
		80%	$2.73
	High	100%	$3.85
		90%	$3.47
		80%	$3.08
	Low	100%	$2.97
		90%	$2.67
		80%	$2.38

LEGEND

	Utilization Levels		
	National	High	Low
Annual Inpatient Days/1000	33	43	26
Annual Inpatient Visits/1000	41	54	32
AnnualOutpatient Visits/1000	300	410	245
	Cost Levels		
	National	High	Low
Cost per Inpatient Day	$850	$1,000	$700
Cost per Inpatient Visit	$80	$85	$75
Cost per Outpatient Visit	$75	$80	$70

No explicit margins or allowances for administrative expenses, coordination of benefits, stop loss reinsurance, adverse risks, or margins for profits and/or contingencies beyond those implicitly provided within the average costs per unit of service have been used.

Medicare Population Capitation Rates
Moderately Managed Care, Inpatient and Outpatient
Copayments: $500 per I/P Admit, $10 per Visit

Utilization Level	Cost Level	% of Medicare Allowable	PMPM Rate
National	National	100%	$4.06
		90%	$3.65
		80%	$3.25
	High	100%	$4.61
		90%	$4.15
		80%	$3.69
	Low	100%	$3.50
		90%	$3.15
		80%	$2.80
High	National	100%	$5.43
		90%	$4.88
		80%	$4.34
	High	100%	$6.16
		90%	$5.54
		80%	$4.93
	Low	100%	$4.69
		90%	$4.23
		80%	$3.76
Low	National	100%	$3.23
		90%	$2.91
		80%	$2.59
	High	100%	$3.68
		90%	$3.31
		80%	$2.94
	Low	100%	$2.79
		90%	$2.51
		80%	$2.24

LEGEND

	Utilization Levels		
	National	High	Low
Annual Inpatient Days/1000	33	43	26
Annual Inpatient Visits/1000	41	54	32
AnnualOutpatient Visits/1000	300	410	245
	Cost Levels		
	National	High	Low
Cost per Inpatient Day	$850	$1,000	$700
Cost per Inpatient Visit	$80	$85	$75
Cost per Outpatient Visit	$75	$80	$70

No explicit margins or allowances for administrative expenses, coordination of benefits, stop loss reinsurance, adverse risks, or margins for profits and/or contingencies beyond those implicitly provided within the average costs per unit of service have been used.

Medicare Population Capitation Rates
Aggressively Managed Care, Inpatient Only
Copayments: None

Utilization Level	Cost Level	% of Medicare Allowable	PMPM Rate
National	National	100%	$4.33
		90%	$3.89
		80%	$3.46
	High	100%	$4.76
		90%	$4.29
		80%	$3.81
	Low	100%	$3.89
		90%	$3.50
		80%	$3.11
High	National	100%	$5.82
		90%	$5.24
		80%	$4.65
	High	100%	$6.40
		90%	$5.76
		80%	$5.12
	Low	100%	$5.24
		90%	$4.71
		80%	$4.19
Low	National	100%	$3.47
		90%	$3.12
		80%	$2.78
	High	100%	$3.85
		90%	$3.46
		80%	$3.08
	Low	100%	$3.09
		90%	$2.78
		80%	$2.47

LEGEND

	Utilization Levels		
	National	High	Low
Annual Inpatient Days/1000	19	25	19
Annual Inpatient Visits/1000	28	36	28
AnnualOutpatient Visits/1000	447	609	310

	Cost Levels		
	National	High	Low
Cost per Inpatient Day	$850	$1,000	$700
Cost per Inpatient Visit	$80	$85	$75
Cost per Outpatient Visit	$75	$80	$70

No explicit margins or allowances for administrative expenses, coordination of benefits, stop loss reinsurance, adverse risks, or margins for profits and/or contingencies beyond those implicitly provided within the average costs per unit of service have been used.

Medicare Population Capitation Rates
Aggressively Managed Care, Inpatient Only
Copayments: $250 per I/P Admit, $5 per Visit

Utilization Level	Cost Level	% of Medicare Allowable	PMPM Rate
National	National	100%	$4.08
		90%	$3.68
		80%	$3.27
	High	100%	$4.52
		90%	$4.07
		80%	$3.62
	Low	100%	$3.65
		90%	$3.28
		80%	$2.92
High	National	100%	$5.50
		90%	$4.95
		80%	$4.40
	High	100%	$6.08
		90%	$5.48
		80%	$4.87
	Low	100%	$4.92
		90%	$4.43
		80%	$3.94
Low	National	100%	$3.28
		90%	$2.96
		80%	$2.63
	High	100%	$3.66
		90%	$3.30
		80%	$2.93
	Low	100%	$2.91
		90%	$2.62
		80%	$2.32

LEGEND

	Utilization Levels		
	National	High	Low
Annual Inpatient Days/1000	19	25	19
Annual Inpatient Visits/1000	28	36	28
AnnualOutpatient Visits/1000	447	609	310

	Cost Levels		
	National	High	Low
Cost per Inpatient Day	$850	$1,000	$700
Cost per Inpatient Visit	$80	$85	$75
Cost per Outpatient Visit	$75	$80	$70

No explicit margins or allowances for administrative expenses, coordination of benefits, stop loss reinsurance, adverse risks, or margins for profits and/or contingencies beyond those implicitly provided within the average costs per unit of service have been used.

Medicare Population Capitation Rates
Aggressively Managed Care, Inpatient Only
Copayments: $500 per I/P Admit, $10 per Visit

Utilization Level	Cost Level	% of Medicare Allowable	PMPM Rate
National	National	100%	$3.84
		90%	$3.46
		80%	$3.07
	High	100%	$4.28
		90%	$3.85
		80%	$3.42
	Low	100%	$3.41
		90%	$3.06
		80%	$2.72
High	National	100%	$5.19
		90%	$4.67
		80%	$4.15
	High	100%	$5.77
		90%	$5.19
		80%	$4.62
	Low	100%	$4.61
		90%	$4.15
		80%	$3.69
Low	National	100%	$3.10
		90%	$2.79
		80%	$2.48
	High	100%	$3.48
		90%	$3.13
		80%	$2.78
	Low	100%	$2.72
		90%	$2.45
		80%	$2.18

LEGEND

	Utilization Levels		
	National	High	Low
Annual Inpatient Days/1000	19	25	19
Annual Inpatient Visits/1000	28	36	28
AnnualOutpatient Visits/1000	447	609	310

	Cost Levels		
	National	High	Low
Cost per Inpatient Day	$850	$1,000	$700
Cost per Inpatient Visit	$80	$85	$75
Cost per Outpatient Visit	$75	$80	$70

No explicit margins or allowances for administrative expenses, coordination of benefits, stop loss reinsurance, adverse risks, or margins for profits and/or contingencies beyond those implicitly provided within the average costs per unit of service have been used.

Medicare Population Capitation Rates
Aggressively Managed Care, Inpatient and Outpatient
Copayments: None

Utilization Level	Cost Level	% of Medicare Allowable	PMPM Rate
National	National	100%	$2.93
		90%	$2.63
		80%	$2.34
	High	100%	$3.27
		90%	$2.94
		80%	$2.61
	Low	100%	$2.58
		90%	$2.33
		80%	$2.07
High	National	100%	$3.92
		90%	$3.53
		80%	$3.13
	High	100%	$4.37
		90%	$3.93
		80%	$3.50
	Low	100%	$3.46
		90%	$3.12
		80%	$2.77
Low	National	100%	$2.93
		90%	$2.63
		80%	$2.34
	High	100%	$3.27
		90%	$2.94
		80%	$2.61
	Low	100%	$2.58
		90%	$2.33
		80%	$2.07

LEGEND

Utilization Levels	National	High	Low
Annual Inpatient Days/1000	19	25	19
Annual Inpatient Visits/1000	28	36	28
AnnualOutpatient Visits/1000	223	305	223

Cost Levels	National	High	Low
Cost per Inpatient Day	$850	$1,000	$700
Cost per Inpatient Visit	$80	$85	$75
Cost per Outpatient Visit	$75	$80	$70

No explicit margins or allowances for administrative expenses, coordination of benefits, stop loss reinsurance, adverse risks, or margins for profits and/or contingencies beyond those implicitly provided within the average costs per unit of service have been used.

Medicare Population Capitation Rates
Aggressively Managed Care, Inpatient and Outpatient
Copayments: $250 per I/P Admit, $5 per Visit

Utilization Level	Cost Level	% of Medicare Allowable	PMPM Rate
National	National	100%	$2.78
		90%	$2.50
		80%	$2.22
	High	100%	$3.12
		90%	$2.81
		80%	$2.50
	Low	100%	$2.43
		90%	$2.19
		80%	$1.95
High	National	100%	$3.73
		90%	$3.36
		80%	$2.98
	High	100%	$4.18
		90%	$3.77
		80%	$3.35
	Low	100%	$3.28
		90%	$2.95
		80%	$2.62
Low	National	100%	$2.78
		90%	$2.50
		80%	$2.22
	High	100%	$3.12
		90%	$2.81
		80%	$2.50
	Low	100%	$2.43
		90%	$2.19
		80%	$1.95

LEGEND

	Utilization Levels		
	National	High	Low
Annual Inpatient Days/1000	19	25	19
Annual Inpatient Visits/1000	28	36	28
AnnualOutpatient Visits/1000	223	305	223
	Cost Levels		
	National	High	Low
Cost per Inpatient Day	$850	$1,000	$700
Cost per Inpatient Visit	$80	$85	$75
Cost per Outpatient Visit	$75	$80	$70

No explicit margins or allowances for administrative expenses, coordination of benefits, stop loss reinsurance, adverse risks, or margins for profits and/or contingencies beyond those implicitly provided within the average costs per unit of service have been used.

Medicare Population Capitation Rates
Aggressively Managed Care, Inpatient and Outpatient
Copayments: $500 per I/P Admit, $10 per Visit

Utilization Level	Cost Level	% of Medicare Allowable	PMPM Rate
National	National	100%	$2.63
		90%	$2.36
		80%	$2.10
	High	100%	$2.97
		90%	$2.67
		80%	$2.38
	Low	100%	$2.29
		90%	$2.06
		80%	$1.83
High	National	100%	$3.54
		90%	$3.19
		80%	$2.83
	High	100%	$4.00
		90%	$3.60
		80%	$3.20
	Low	100%	$3.09
		90%	$2.78
		80%	$2.47
Low	National	100%	$2.63
		90%	$2.36
		80%	$2.10
	High	100%	$2.97
		90%	$2.67
		80%	$2.38
	Low	100%	$2.29
		90%	$2.06
		80%	$1.83

LEGEND

Utilization Levels	National	High	Low
Annual Inpatient Days/1000	19	25	19
Annual Inpatient Visits/1000	28	36	28
AnnualOutpatient Visits/1000	223	305	223

Cost Levels	National	High	Low
Cost per Inpatient Day	$850	$1,000	$700
Cost per Inpatient Visit	$80	$85	$75
Cost per Outpatient Visit	$75	$80	$70

No explicit margins or allowances for administrative expenses, coordination of benefits, stop loss reinsurance, adverse risks, or margins for profits and/or contingencies beyond those implicitly provided within the average costs per unit of service have been used.

The preceding tables can be used to develop capitation estimates for various combinations of ·

- ♦ **Degree of Managed Care**—Unmanaged vs. Moderately Managed vs. Aggressively Managed, Inpatient Only vs. Inpatient and Outpatient Management
- ♦ **Utilization Level Before Application of Managed Care**—National vs. High (about 130%–135% of National) vs. Low (about 70% of National)
- ♦ **Cost Level**—National vs. High (about 120%–125% of National) vs. Low (about 75%–80% of National)
- ♦ **Discount to Medicare Allowable Levels**—no discount vs. 20% discount vs. 40% discount
- ♦ **Benefit Plan Copayments**—None vs. $250 per inpatient admit/$5 per professional visit vs. $500 per inpatient admit/$10 per professional visit

For example, a Medicare population behavioral healthcare capitation offer of $4.00 per member per month would be adequate for expected benefit costs for the following different scenarios:

	Scenario 1	Scenario 2	Scenario 3
Degree of Managed Care	Unmanaged	Moderate-I/P and O/P	Aggressive I/P and O/P
Utilization Level	Low	National	High
Cost Level	High	National	National
Discount to Medicare Allowable	20%	10%	None
Copayments	$250 per I/P admit	$250 per I/P admit	None
	$5 per visit	$5 per visit	None

However, little additional margin would exist for administrative expenses, adverse risks, profits, etc., beyond those implicitly provided within the average costs per unit of service. If higher utilization levels, higher cost levels, smaller discounts to Medicare allowable charge levels, or lesser degrees of managed care were expected (without any offsetting factors), the $4.00 PMPM capitation rate may be inadequate. Conversely, if lower utilization levels, lower cost levels, larger discounts to Medicare allowable charge levels, or higher degrees of managed care were expected (without any offsetting factors), the $4.00 PMPM capitation rate would provide additional sources of profits or margins for expenses and/or other contingencies.

Capitation Rates for the Medicaid Population

X.   CAPITATION RATES FOR THE MEDICAID POPULATION

Capitation under Medicaid managed care programs is expanding, with Medicaid full-risk HMO enrollment being significantly higher in states with high private sector HMO enrollment. There are many variables applicable to the Medicaid population that make cost estimates for behavioral health-care more difficult than the commercially insured and Medicare populations.

- Medicaid eligible groups can vary significantly from state to state, and between urban and rural areas.
- The composition of the categorically needy can greatly impact the over-all Medicaid costs per member.

  - SSI recipients can cost five times or more than AFDC recipients.
  - Foster care children (out-of-home placements who meet income and eligibility requirements) can cost twenty-five times or more than AFDC recipients.

- The non-cash Medicaid population can vary dramatically from state to state.
- Behavioral healthcare benefits to the Medicaid population can vary by state.
- The continuum of care available to the Medicaid population can vary by state and locale.
- The composition of the professional providers available and willing to serve the Medicaid population can vary by state and locale, affecting average unit costs by type of service.
- The amount and degree of case management services (specification and management of behavioral health care treatment plans and potentially some social and maintenance services) can vary by state and locale.
- The amount of psychosocial services (rehabilitation, home and community services, community health, etc.) can vary by state and locale.

We have incorporated these variables within our Medicaid behavioral healthcare cost estimates by using the following:

- Three different utilization scenarios for aggregate inpatient and outpatient services
- Ranges of utilization rates per 1,000 covered members within each utilization scenario, with corresponding ranges of per member per month cost estimates
- Three different average unit cost levels for facilities and professional services

♦ Three different aggregate per member per month cost levels for case management services

The following table presents our Medicaid behavioral healthcare cost estimates for the various scenarios described above. The distribution of Medicaid eligibles that is consistent with these cost estimates is approximately 72% AFDC, 27% SSI (aged, blind, disabled) and 1% Foster Care.

No explicit margins or allowances for administrative expenses, coordination of benefits, stop loss reinsurance, adverse risks, or margins for profits and/or contingencies beyond those implicitly provided within the average costs per unit of service have been used. The costs also do <u>not</u> include psychosocial costs.

Medicaid Capitation Scenarios

Utilization Scenario	Cost Scenario	Annual Facility Utilization per 1,000	Facility Cost/ Day	Annual Professional Utilization per 1,000	Professional Cost/Visit	Case Management PMPM Cost	PMPM Rate
High	High	450–500	$500	3000–3250	$60	$2.50	$36.25–$39.58
	Mid	450–500	$400	3000–3250	$50	$2.00	$29.50–$32.21
	Low	450–500	$300	3000–3250	$40	$1.50	$22.75–$24.83
Mid	High	300–350	$500	2000–2250	$60	$2.00	$24.50–$27.83
	Mid	300–350	$400	2000–2250	$50	$1.60	$19.93–$22.64
	Low	300–350	$300	2000–2250	$40	$1.20	$15.37–$17.45
Low	High	150–200	$500	1000–1250	$60	$1.50	$12.75–$16.08
	Mid	150–200	$400	1000–1250	$50	$1.25	$10.42–$13.13
	Low	150–200	$300	1000–1250	$40	$1.00	$8.08–$10.17

No explicit margins or allowances for administrative expenses, coordination of benefits, stop loss reinsurance, adverse risks, or margins for profits and/or contingencies beyond those implicitly provided within the average costs per unit of service have been used.

The three different utilization scenarios can be used to differentiate between high, mid, and low user Medicaid populations and/or to differentiate between managed care utilization levels. For a given average Medicaid population, the high utilization level is consistent with unmanaged or more loosely managed behavioral healthcare, the mid utilization level is consistent with moderate levels of managed delivery, while the low utilization level is reflective of more aggressively managed delivery system.

Ranges of utilization rates are used, together with ranges of ultimate corresponding PMPM costs, to reflect the higher level of uncertainty associated with the Medicaid population as compared to the commercially insured population.

The above table can be used to develop capitation estimates given a level of utilization and unit costs, or to develop required utilization and/or cost levels given a capitation offer. For example, an aggregate Medicaid behavioral healthcare capitation offer of $25 per member per month could support mid-level utilization (300–350 annual facility days per 1,000 and 2,0002,250 annual professional visits per 1,000 members), **mid-level unit costs ($400 per facility day and $50 per professional visit), mid-level case management costs ($1.60 PMPM), and a margin of 10% for administrative expenses, stoploss reinsurance, adverse risks and profits. If higher utilization and/or unit costs were expected, the capitation may be inadequate. However, if lower utilization and/or unit cost levels could be achieved, the capitation offer is projected to be more than adequate, providing additional sources of profits or margins for expenses and/or other contingencies.**

If psychosocial services are provided to the Medicaid population, an explicit cost PMPM should be added for such services.

APPENDIXES

DETAILED RESULTS FOR THE COMMERCIAL POPULATION, SORTED BY CAPITATION RATE

We developed capitation rates in this report by applying actuarial relationships among benefit limits, local costs, degree of healthcare management, patient cost sharing, and provider discounts for ADM services. Certain combinations of these factors (e.g., low benefit plans combined with low local cost levels, aggressive care management, high patient cost sharing, and large provider discounts) produce low capitation rates. We recognize the APA's concerns that overly low capitation rates simply may not allow physicians to provide an adequate amount of care. Certainly, poor quality or poor access can occur in plans that appear to offer generous benefits or reimbursement. We do not intend for this report to be used by organizations to justify inadequate capitation rates for ADM providers. Rather, we present rates associated with these various combinations of factors in order to provide general guidance and education to APA members on these capitation issues.

Appendix I
Commercial Population Capitation Rates Sorted by Scenario Rate
PMPM Capitation Payments by Scenario
Estimated Psych & Substance Abuse Claim Costs as of July 1, 1995

Plan Type	Area Cost	Copay Level	Management Type	Discount Level
Capitation at least $13.00 but less than $17.00				
Unlimited IP Days, IP Visits, OP Visits	National Avg. + 20%	$0 per Admit, $10 per OP Visit	Loosely Managed (Unmanaged)	20%
Unlimited IP Days, IP Visits, OP Visits	National Avg. + 20%	$200 per Admit, $25 per OP Visit	Loosely Managed (Unmanaged)	20%
Unlimited IP Days, IP Visits, OP Visits	National Avg. + 20%	$0 per Admit, $10 per OP Visit	Loosely Managed (Unmanaged)	30%
Unlimited IP Days, IP Visits, OP Visits	National Avg. + 20%	$0 per Admit, $10 per OP Visit	Moderately Managed - I/P Only	20%
Unlimited IP Days, IP Visits, OP Visits	National Avg.	$0 per Admit, $10 per OP Visit	Loosely Managed (Unmanaged)	20%
45 IP Days, 45 IP Visits, 30 OP Visits	National Avg. + 20%	$0 per Admit, $10 per OP Visit	Loosely Managed (Unmanaged)	20%
Unlimited IP Days, IP Visits, OP Visits	National Avg. + 20%	$200 per Admit, $25 per OP Visit	Loosely Managed (Unmanaged)	30%
Capitation at least $12.00 but less than $13.00				
Unlimited IP Days, IP Visits, OP Visits	National Avg. + 20%	$0 per Admit, $10 per OP Visit	Loosely Managed (Unmanaged)	40%
Unlimited IP Days, IP Visits, OP Visits	National Avg.	$200 per Admit, $25 per OP Visit	Loosely Managed (Unmanaged)	20%
45 IP Days, 45 IP Visits, 30 OP Visits	National Avg. + 20%	$200 per Admit, $25 per OP Visit	Loosely Managed (Unmanaged)	20%
30 IP Days, 30 IP Visits, 20 OP Visits	National Avg. + 20%	$0 per Admit, $10 per OP Visit	Loosely Managed (Unmanaged)	20%
Unlimited IP Days, IP Visits, OP Visits	National Avg. + 20%	$200 per Admit, $25 per OP Visit	Moderately Managed - I/P Only	20%
Capitation at least $11.00 but less than $12.00				
Unlimited IP Days, IP Visits, OP Visits	National Avg. + 20%	$0 per Admit, $10 per OP Visit	Moderately Managed - I/P & O/P	20%
Unlimited IP Days, IP Visits, OP Visits	National Avg.	$0 per Admit, $10 per OP Visit	Loosely Managed (Unmanaged)	30%
Unlimited IP Days, IP Visits, OP Visits	National Avg. + 20%	$0 per Admit, $10 per OP Visit	Moderately Managed - I/P Only	30%
45 IP Days, 45 IP Visits, 30 OP Visits	National Avg. + 20%	$0 per Admit, $10 per OP Visit	Loosely Managed (Unmanaged)	30%
Unlimited IP Days, IP Visits, OP Visits	National Avg. + 20%	$200 per Admit, $25 per OP Visit	Loosely Managed (Unmanaged)	40%
30 IP Days, 30 IP Visits, 20 OP Visits	National Avg. + 20%	$200 per Admit, $25 per OP Visit	Loosely Managed (Unmanaged)	20%
45 IP Days, 45 IP Visits, 30 OP Visits	National Avg. + 20%	$0 per Admit, $10 per OP Visit	Moderately Managed - I/P Only	20%
Unlimited IP Days, IP Visits, OP Visits	National Avg.	$0 per Admit, $10 per OP Visit	Moderately Managed - I/P Only	20%
15 IP Days, 15 IP Visits, 45 OP Visits	National Avg. + 20%	$0 per Admit, $10 per OP Visit	Loosely Managed (Unmanaged)	20%
Capitation at least $10.00 but less than $11.00				
45 IP Days, 45 IP Visits, 30 OP Visits	National Avg.	$0 per Admit, $10 per OP Visit	Loosely Managed (Unmanaged)	20%
Unlimited IP Days, IP Visits, OP Visits	National Avg. - 20%	$0 per Admit, $10 per OP Visit	Loosely Managed (Unmanaged)	20%
Unlimited IP Days, IP Visits, OP Visits	National Avg.	$200 per Admit, $25 per OP Visit	Loosely Managed (Unmanaged)	30%
Unlimited IP Days, IP Visits, OP Visits	National Avg. + 20%	$200 per Admit, $25 per OP Visit	Moderately Managed - I/P & O/P	20%
30 IP Days, 30 IP Visits, 20 OP Visits	National Avg. + 20%	$0 per Admit, $10 per OP Visit	Loosely Managed (Unmanaged)	30%
45 IP Days, 45 IP Visits, 30 OP Visits	National Avg. + 20%	$200 per Admit, $25 per OP Visit	Loosely Managed (Unmanaged)	30%
Unlimited IP Days, IP Visits, OP Visits	National Avg. + 20%	$0 per Admit, $10 per OP Visit	Aggressively Managed - I/P Only	20%
Unlimited IP Days, IP Visits, OP Visits	National Avg. + 20%	$200 per Admit, $25 per OP Visit	Moderately Managed - I/P Only	30%
Unlimited IP Days, IP Visits, OP Visits	National Avg. + 20%	$0 per Admit, $10 per OP Visit	Moderately Managed - I/P & O/P	30%
Unlimited IP Days, IP Visits, OP Visits	National Avg.	$0 per Admit, $10 per OP Visit	Loosely Managed (Unmanaged)	40%
Capitation at least $9.50 but less than $10.00				
Unlimited IP Days, IP Visits, OP Visits	National Avg. + 20%	$0 per Admit, $10 per OP Visit	Moderately Managed - I/P Only	40%
30 IP Days, 30 IP Visits, 20 OP Visits	National Avg. + 20%	$0 per Admit, $10 per OP Visit	Moderately Managed - I/P Only	20%
45 IP Days, 45 IP Visits, 30 OP Visits	National Avg. + 20%	$0 per Admit, $10 per OP Visit	Loosely Managed (Unmanaged)	40%
15 IP Days, 15 IP Visits, 45 OP Visits	National Avg. + 20%	$0 per Admit, $10 per OP Visit	Moderately Managed - I/P Only	20%
30 IP Days, 30 IP Visits, 20 OP Visits	National Avg.	$0 per Admit, $10 per OP Visit	Loosely Managed (Unmanaged)	20%
45 IP Days, 45 IP Visits, 30 OP Visits	National Avg.	$200 per Admit, $25 per OP Visit	Loosely Managed (Unmanaged)	20%
15 IP Days, 15 IP Visits, 45 OP Visits	National Avg. + 20%	$200 per Admit, $25 per OP Visit	Loosely Managed (Unmanaged)	20%
Unlimited IP Days, IP Visits, OP Visits	National Avg. - 20%	$200 per Admit, $25 per OP Visit	Loosely Managed (Unmanaged)	20%
45 IP Days, 45 IP Visits, 30 OP Visits	National Avg. + 20%	$200 per Admit, $25 per OP Visit	Moderately Managed - I/P Only	20%
Unlimited IP Days, IP Visits, OP Visits	National Avg.	$200 per Admit, $25 per OP Visit	Moderately Managed - I/P Only	20%
30 IP Days, 30 IP Visits, 20 OP Visits	National Avg. + 20%	$200 per Admit, $25 per OP Visit	Loosely Managed (Unmanaged)	30%
Unlimited IP Days, IP Visits, OP Visits	National Avg.	$0 per Admit, $10 per OP Visit	Moderately Managed - I/P & O/P	20%

No explicit margins or allowances for administrative expenses, coordination of benefits, stop loss reinsurance, adverse risks, or margins for profits and/or contingencies beyond those implicitly provided within the average costs per unit of service have been used.

Appendix I
Commercial Population Capitation Rates Sorted by Scenario Rate
PMPM Capitation Payments by Scenario
Estimated Psych & Substance Abuse Claim Costs as of July 1, 1995

Plan Type	Area Cost	Copay Level	Management Type	Discount Level
Capitation at least $9.00 but less than $9.50				
45 IP Days, 45 IP Visits, 30 OP Visits	National Avg. + 20%	$0 per Admit, $10 per OP Visit	Moderately Managed - I/P & O/P	20%
Unlimited IP Days, IP Visits, OP Visits	National Avg.	$0 per Admit, $10 per OP Visit	Moderately Managed - I/P Only	30%
45 IP Days, 45 IP Visits, 30 OP Visits	National Avg. + 20%	$0 per Admit, $10 per OP Visit	Moderately Managed - I/P Only	30%
15 IP Days, 15 IP Visits, 45 OP Visits	National Avg. + 20%	$0 per Admit, $10 per OP Visit	Loosely Managed (Unmanaged)	30%
15 IP Days, 15 IP Visits, 45 OP Visits	National Avg. + 20%	$0 per Admit, $10 per OP Visit	Aggressively Managed - I/P Only	20%
45 IP Days, 45 IP Visits, 30 OP Visits	National Avg.	$0 per Admit, $10 per OP Visit	Loosely Managed (Unmanaged)	30%
Unlimited IP Days, IP Visits, OP Visits	National Avg. - 20%	$0 per Admit, $10 per OP Visit	Loosely Managed (Unmanaged)	30%
Unlimited IP Days, IP Visits, OP Visits	National Avg. + 20%	$200 per Admit, $25 per OP Visit	Moderately Managed - I/P & O/P	30%
Capitation at least $8.50 but less than $9.00				
30 IP Days, 30 IP Visits, 20 OP Visits	National Avg. + 20%	$0 per Admit, $10 per OP Visit	Loosely Managed (Unmanaged)	40%
45 IP Days, 45 IP Visits, 30 OP Visits	National Avg.	$0 per Admit, $10 per OP Visit	Moderately Managed - I/P Only	20%
30 IP Days, 30 IP Visits, 20 OP Visits	National Avg.	$200 per Admit, $25 per OP Visit	Loosely Managed (Unmanaged)	20%
Unlimited IP Days, IP Visits, OP Visits	National Avg.	$200 per Admit, $25 per OP Visit	Loosely Managed (Unmanaged)	40%
15 IP Days, 15 IP Visits, 45 OP Visits	National Avg.	$0 per Admit, $10 per OP Visit	Loosely Managed (Unmanaged)	20%
Unlimited IP Days, IP Visits, OP Visits	National Avg. + 20%	$0 per Admit, $10 per OP Visit	Aggressively Managed - I/P Only	30%
45 IP Days, 45 IP Visits, 30 OP Visits	National Avg. + 20%	$200 per Admit, $25 per OP Visit	Loosely Managed (Unmanaged)	40%
Unlimited IP Days, IP Visits, OP Visits	National Avg. - 20%	$0 per Admit, $10 per OP Visit	Moderately Managed - I/P Only	20%
45 IP Days, 45 IP Visits, 30 OP Visits	National Avg. + 20%	$0 per Admit, $10 per OP Visit	Aggressively Managed - I/P Only	20%
30 IP Days, 30 IP Visits, 20 OP Visits	National Avg. + 20%	$200 per Admit, $25 per OP Visit	Moderately Managed - I/P Only	20%
Unlimited IP Days, IP Visits, OP Visits	National Avg. + 20%	$0 per Admit, $10 per OP Visit	Moderately Managed - I/P & O/P	40%
Unlimited IP Days, IP Visits, OP Visits	National Avg. + 20%	$200 per Admit, $25 per OP Visit	Aggressively Managed - I/P Only	20%
30 IP Days, 30 IP Visits, 20 OP Visits	National Avg. + 20%	$0 per Admit, $10 per OP Visit	Moderately Managed - I/P & O/P	20%
45 IP Days, 45 IP Visits, 30 OP Visits	National Avg. - 20%	$0 per Admit, $10 per OP Visit	Loosely Managed (Unmanaged)	20%
Unlimited IP Days, IP Visits, OP Visits	National Avg.	$200 per Admit, $25 per OP Visit	Moderately Managed - I/P & O/P	20%
Unlimited IP Days, IP Visits, OP Visits	National Avg.	$0 per Admit, $10 per OP Visit	Aggressively Managed - I/P Only	20%
Capitation at least $8.00 but less than $8.50				
30 IP Days, 30 IP Visits, 20 OP Visits	National Avg. + 20%	$0 per Admit, $10 per OP Visit	Moderately Managed - I/P Only	30%
30 IP Days, 30 IP Visits, 20 OP Visits	National Avg.	$0 per Admit, $10 per OP Visit	Loosely Managed (Unmanaged)	30%
45 IP Days, 45 IP Visits, 30 OP Visits	National Avg. + 20%	$200 per Admit, $25 per OP Visit	Moderately Managed - I/P & O/P	20%
Unlimited IP Days, IP Visits, OP Visits	National Avg. + 20%	$200 per Admit, $25 per OP Visit	Moderately Managed - I/P Only	40%
15 IP Days, 15 IP Visits, 45 OP Visits	National Avg. + 20%	$0 per Admit, $10 per OP Visit	Moderately Managed - I/P Only	30%
45 IP Days, 45 IP Visits, 30 OP Visits	National Avg.	$200 per Admit, $25 per OP Visit	Loosely Managed (Unmanaged)	30%
15 IP Days, 15 IP Visits, 45 OP Visits	National Avg. + 20%	$200 per Admit, $25 per OP Visit	Moderately Managed - I/P Only	20%
Unlimited IP Days, IP Visits, OP Visits	National Avg. - 20%	$200 per Admit, $25 per OP Visit	Loosely Managed (Unmanaged)	30%
15 IP Days, 15 IP Visits, 45 OP Visits	National Avg. + 20%	$200 per Admit, $25 per OP Visit	Loosely Managed (Unmanaged)	30%
Unlimited IP Days, IP Visits, OP Visits	National Avg.	$0 per Admit, $10 per OP Visit	Moderately Managed - I/P & O/P	30%
45 IP Days, 45 IP Visits, 30 OP Visits	National Avg. + 20%	$200 per Admit, $25 per OP Visit	Moderately Managed - I/P Only	30%
45 IP Days, 45 IP Visits, 30 OP Visits	National Avg. + 20%	$0 per Admit, $10 per OP Visit	Moderately Managed - I/P & O/P	30%
Unlimited IP Days, IP Visits, OP Visits	National Avg.	$200 per Admit, $25 per OP Visit	Moderately Managed - I/P Only	30%
15 IP Days, 15 IP Visits, 45 OP Visits	National Avg. + 20%	$0 per Admit, $10 per OP Visit	Moderately Managed - I/P & O/P	20%
45 IP Days, 45 IP Visits, 30 OP Visits	National Avg. + 20%	$0 per Admit, $10 per OP Visit	Moderately Managed - I/P Only	40%
Unlimited IP Days, IP Visits, OP Visits	National Avg.	$0 per Admit, $10 per OP Visit	Moderately Managed - I/P Only	40%
15 IP Days, 15 IP Visits, 45 OP Visits	National Avg.	$0 per Admit, $10 per OP Visit	Moderately Managed - I/P Only	20%
15 IP Days, 15 IP Visits, 45 OP Visits	National Avg. + 20%	$0 per Admit, $10 per OP Visit	Loosely Managed (Unmanaged)	40%
30 IP Days, 30 IP Visits, 20 OP Visits	National Avg.	$0 per Admit, $10 per OP Visit	Moderately Managed - I/P Only	20%

No explicit margins or allowances for administrative expenses, coordination of benefits, stop loss reinsurance, adverse risks, or margins for profits and/or contingencies beyond those implicitly provided within the average costs per unit of service have been used.

Appendix I
Commercial Population Capitation Rates Sorted by Scenario Rate
PMPM Capitation Payments by Scenario
Estimated Psych & Substance Abuse Claim Costs as of July 1, 1995

Plan Type	Area Cost	Copay Level	Management Type	Discount Level
Capitation at least $7.50 but less than $8.00				
30 IP Days, 30 IP Visits, 20 OP Visits	National Avg. + 20%	$200 per Admit, $25 per OP Visit	Loosely Managed (Unmanaged)	40%
45 IP Days, 45 IP Visits, 30 OP Visits	National Avg.	$0 per Admit, $10 per OP Visit	Loosely Managed (Unmanaged)	40%
Unlimited IP Days, IP Visits, OP Visits	National Avg. - 20%	$0 per Admit, $10 per OP Visit	Loosely Managed (Unmanaged)	40%
15 IP Days, 15 IP Visits, 45 OP Visits	National Avg. + 20%	$0 per Admit, $10 per OP Visit	Aggressively Managed - I/P Only	30%
15 IP Days, 15 IP Visits, 45 OP Visits	National Avg.	$200 per Admit, $25 per OP Visit	Loosely Managed (Unmanaged)	20%
45 IP Days, 45 IP Visits, 30 OP Visits	National Avg.	$200 per Admit, $25 per OP Visit	Moderately Managed - I/P Only	20%
30 IP Days, 30 IP Visits, 20 OP Visits	National Avg. + 20%	$0 per Admit, $10 per OP Visit	Aggressively Managed - I/P Only	20%
30 IP Days, 30 IP Visits, 20 OP Visits	National Avg. - 20%	$0 per Admit, $10 per OP Visit	Loosely Managed (Unmanaged)	20%
15 IP Days, 15 IP Visits, 45 OP Visits	National Avg.	$0 per Admit, $10 per OP Visit	Aggressively Managed - I/P Only	20%
45 IP Days, 45 IP Visits, 30 OP Visits	National Avg.	$0 per Admit, $10 per OP Visit	Moderately Managed - I/P & O/P	20%
45 IP Days, 45 IP Visits, 30 OP Visits	National Avg.	$0 per Admit, $10 per OP Visit	Moderately Managed - I/P Only	30%
45 IP Days, 45 IP Visits, 30 OP Visits	National Avg. - 20%	$200 per Admit, $25 per OP Visit	Loosely Managed (Unmanaged)	20%
30 IP Days, 30 IP Visits, 20 OP Visits	National Avg. + 20%	$200 per Admit, $25 per OP Visit	Moderately Managed - I/P & O/P	20%
15 IP Days, 15 IP Visits, 45 OP Visits	National Avg.	$0 per Admit, $10 per OP Visit	Loosely Managed (Unmanaged)	30%
30 IP Days, 30 IP Visits, 20 OP Visits	National Avg.	$200 per Admit, $25 per OP Visit	Loosely Managed (Unmanaged)	30%
15 IP Days, 15 IP Visits, 45 OP Visits	National Avg. + 20%	$200 per Admit, $25 per OP Visit	Aggressively Managed - I/P Only	20%
Unlimited IP Days, IP Visits, OP Visits	National Avg. - 20%	$0 per Admit, $10 per OP Visit	Moderately Managed - I/P Only	30%
Unlimited IP Days, IP Visits, OP Visits	National Avg. - 20%	$200 per Admit, $25 per OP Visit	Moderately Managed - I/P Only	20%
Unlimited IP Days, IP Visits, OP Visits	National Avg. + 20%	$200 per Admit, $25 per OP Visit	Moderately Managed - I/P & O/P	40%
Unlimited IP Days, IP Visits, OP Visits	National Avg. - 20%	$0 per Admit, $10 per OP Visit	Moderately Managed - I/P & O/P	20%
Capitation at least $7.00 but less than $7.50				
Unlimited IP Days, IP Visits, OP Visits	National Avg. + 20%	$0 per Admit, $10 per OP Visit	Aggressively Managed - I/P Only	40%
45 IP Days, 45 IP Visits, 30 OP Visits	National Avg. - 20%	$0 per Admit, $10 per OP Visit	Loosely Managed (Unmanaged)	30%
45 IP Days, 45 IP Visits, 30 OP Visits	National Avg. + 20%	$0 per Admit, $10 per OP Visit	Aggressively Managed - I/P Only	30%
30 IP Days, 30 IP Visits, 20 OP Visits	National Avg. + 20%	$200 per Admit, $25 per OP Visit	Moderately Managed - I/P Only	30%
30 IP Days, 30 IP Visits, 20 OP Visits	National Avg. + 20%	$0 per Admit, $10 per OP Visit	Moderately Managed - I/P & O/P	30%
Unlimited IP Days, IP Visits, OP Visits	National Avg.	$200 per Admit, $25 per OP Visit	Moderately Managed - I/P & O/P	30%
30 IP Days, 30 IP Visits, 20 OP Visits	National Avg. + 20%	$0 per Admit, $10 per OP Visit	Moderately Managed - I/P Only	40%
30 IP Days, 30 IP Visits, 20 OP Visits	National Avg.	$0 per Admit, $10 per OP Visit	Loosely Managed (Unmanaged)	40%
45 IP Days, 45 IP Visits, 30 OP Visits	National Avg. + 20%	$200 per Admit, $25 per OP Visit	Moderately Managed - I/P & O/P	30%
Unlimited IP Days, IP Visits, OP Visits	National Avg.	$0 per Admit, $10 per OP Visit	Aggressively Managed - I/P Only	30%
15 IP Days, 15 IP Visits, 45 OP Visits	National Avg. + 20%	$0 per Admit, $10 per OP Visit	Moderately Managed - I/P Only	40%
45 IP Days, 45 IP Visits, 30 OP Visits	National Avg.	$0 per Admit, $10 per OP Visit	Aggressively Managed - I/P Only	20%
45 IP Days, 45 IP Visits, 30 OP Visits	National Avg. - 20%	$0 per Admit, $10 per OP Visit	Moderately Managed - I/P Only	20%
Unlimited IP Days, IP Visits, OP Visits	National Avg. + 20%	$200 per Admit, $25 per OP Visit	Aggressively Managed - I/P Only	30%
45 IP Days, 45 IP Visits, 30 OP Visits	National Avg. + 20%	$200 per Admit, $25 per OP Visit	Aggressively Managed - I/P Only	20%
15 IP Days, 15 IP Visits, 45 OP Visits	National Avg. + 20%	$200 per Admit, $25 per OP Visit	Moderately Managed - I/P & O/P	20%
15 IP Days, 15 IP Visits, 45 OP Visits	National Avg. + 20%	$200 per Admit, $25 per OP Visit	Moderately Managed - I/P Only	30%

No explicit margins or allowances for administrative expenses, coordination of benefits, stop loss reinsurance, adverse risks, or margins for profits and/or contingencies beyond those implicitly provided within the average costs per unit of service have been used.

Appendix I
Commercial Population Capitation Rates Sorted by Scenario Rate
PMPM Capitation Payments by Scenario
Estimated Psych & Substance Abuse Claim Costs as of July 1, 1995

Plan Type	Area Cost	Copay Level	Management Type	Discount Level
Capitation at least $6.50 but less than $7.00				
15 IP Days, 15 IP Visits, 45 OP Visits	National Avg. - 20%	$0 per Admit, $10 per OP Visit	Loosely Managed (Unmanaged)	20%
Unlimited IP Days, IP Visits, OP Visits	National Avg.	$0 per Admit, $10 per OP Visit	Moderately Managed - I/P & O/P	40%
45 IP Days, 45 IP Visits, 30 OP Visits	National Avg.	$200 per Admit, $25 per OP Visit	Loosely Managed (Unmanaged)	40%
30 IP Days, 30 IP Visits, 20 OP Visits	National Avg.	$200 per Admit, $25 per OP Visit	Moderately Managed - I/P Only	20%
30 IP Days, 30 IP Visits, 20 OP Visits	National Avg. - 20%	$200 per Admit, $25 per OP Visit	Loosely Managed (Unmanaged)	20%
15 IP Days, 15 IP Visits, 45 OP Visits	National Avg. + 20%	$0 per Admit, $10 per OP Visit	Moderately Managed - I/P & O/P	30%
45 IP Days, 45 IP Visits, 30 OP Visits	National Avg. + 20%	$0 per Admit, $10 per OP Visit	Moderately Managed - I/P & O/P	40%
Unlimited IP Days, IP Visits, OP Visits	National Avg. - 20%	$200 per Admit, $25 per OP Visit	Loosely Managed (Unmanaged)	40%
30 IP Days, 30 IP Visits, 20 OP Visits	National Avg.	$0 per Admit, $10 per OP Visit	Moderately Managed - I/P & O/P	20%
30 IP Days, 30 IP Visits, 20 OP Visits	National Avg.	$0 per Admit, $10 per OP Visit	Moderately Managed - I/P Only	30%
Unlimited IP Days, IP Visits, OP Visits	National Avg.	$200 per Admit, $25 per OP Visit	Aggressively Managed - I/P Only	20%
15 IP Days, 15 IP Visits, 45 OP Visits	National Avg.	$0 per Admit, $10 per OP Visit	Moderately Managed - I/P Only	30%
15 IP Days, 15 IP Visits, 45 OP Visits	National Avg. + 20%	$200 per Admit, $25 per OP Visit	Loosely Managed (Unmanaged)	40%
45 IP Days, 45 IP Visits, 30 OP Visits	National Avg.	$200 per Admit, $25 per OP Visit	Moderately Managed - I/P & O/P	20%
45 IP Days, 45 IP Visits, 30 OP Visits	National Avg. + 20%	$200 per Admit, $25 per OP Visit	Moderately Managed - I/P Only	40%
30 IP Days, 30 IP Visits, 20 OP Visits	National Avg. - 20%	$0 per Admit, $10 per OP Visit	Loosely Managed (Unmanaged)	30%
Unlimited IP Days, IP Visits, OP Visits	National Avg.	$200 per Admit, $25 per OP Visit	Moderately Managed - I/P Only	40%
Unlimited IP Days, IP Visits, OP Visits	National Avg. - 20%	$0 per Admit, $10 per OP Visit	Aggressively Managed - I/P Only	20%
15 IP Days, 15 IP Visits, 45 OP Visits	National Avg.	$200 per Admit, $25 per OP Visit	Moderately Managed - I/P Only	20%
15 IP Days, 15 IP Visits, 45 OP Visits	National Avg. + 20%	$0 per Admit, $10 per OP Visit	Aggressively Managed - I/P Only	40%
Unlimited IP Days, IP Visits, OP Visits	National Avg. - 20%	$200 per Admit, $25 per OP Visit	Moderately Managed - I/P & O/P	20%
15 IP Days, 15 IP Visits, 45 OP Visits	National Avg.	$0 per Admit, $10 per OP Visit	Moderately Managed - I/P & O/P	20%
45 IP Days, 45 IP Visits, 30 OP Visits	National Avg.	$0 per Admit, $10 per OP Visit	Moderately Managed - I/P & O/P	30%
15 IP Days, 15 IP Visits, 45 OP Visits	National Avg.	$200 per Admit, $25 per OP Visit	Loosely Managed (Unmanaged)	30%
30 IP Days, 30 IP Visits, 20 OP Visits	National Avg. + 20%	$0 per Admit, $10 per OP Visit	Aggressively Managed - I/P Only	30%
45 IP Days, 45 IP Visits, 30 OP Visits	National Avg. - 20%	$200 per Admit, $25 per OP Visit	Loosely Managed (Unmanaged)	30%
Unlimited IP Days, IP Visits, OP Visits	National Avg. - 20%	$0 per Admit, $10 per OP Visit	Moderately Managed - I/P & O/P	30%
45 IP Days, 45 IP Visits, 30 OP Visits	National Avg.	$200 per Admit, $25 per OP Visit	Moderately Managed - I/P Only	30%
45 IP Days, 45 IP Visits, 30 OP Visits	National Avg.	$0 per Admit, $10 per OP Visit	Moderately Managed - I/P Only	40%

No explicit margins or allowances for administrative expenses, coordination of benefits, stop loss reinsurance, adverse risks, or margins for profits and/or contingencies beyond those implicitly provided within the average costs per unit of service have been used.

Appendix I
Commercial Population Capitation Rates Sorted by Scenario Rate
PMPM Capitation Payments by Scenario
Estimated Psych & Substance Abuse Claim Costs as of July 1, 1995

Plan Type	Area Cost	Copay Level	Management Type	Discount Level
Capitation at least $6.00 but less than $6.50				
30 IP Days, 30 IP Visits, 20 OP Visits	National Avg. + 20%	$200 per Admit, $25 per OP Visit	Moderately Managed - I/P & O/P	30%
15 IP Days, 15 IP Visits, 45 OP Visits	National Avg.	$0 per Admit, $10 per OP Visit	Loosely Managed (Unmanaged)	40%
15 IP Days, 15 IP Visits, 45 OP Visits	National Avg.	$0 per Admit, $10 per OP Visit	Aggressively Managed - I/P Only	30%
Unlimited IP Days, IP Visits, OP Visits	National Avg. + 20%	$0 per Admit, $10 per OP Visit	Aggressively Managed - I/P & O/P	20%
Unlimited IP Days, IP Visits, OP Visits	National Avg. - 20%	$0 per Admit, $10 per OP Visit	Moderately Managed - I/P Only	40%
30 IP Days, 30 IP Visits, 20 OP Visits	National Avg.	$200 per Admit, $25 per OP Visit	Loosely Managed (Unmanaged)	40%
30 IP Days, 30 IP Visits, 20 OP Visits	National Avg.	$0 per Admit, $10 per OP Visit	Aggressively Managed - I/P Only	20%
15 IP Days, 15 IP Visits, 45 OP Visits	National Avg. - 20%	$0 per Admit, $10 per OP Visit	Moderately Managed - I/P Only	20%
30 IP Days, 30 IP Visits, 20 OP Visits	National Avg. + 20%	$200 per Admit, $25 per OP Visit	Aggressively Managed - I/P Only	20%
Unlimited IP Days, IP Visits, OP Visits	National Avg. - 20%	$200 per Admit, $25 per OP Visit	Moderately Managed - I/P Only	30%
30 IP Days, 30 IP Visits, 20 OP Visits	National Avg. - 20%	$0 per Admit, $10 per OP Visit	Moderately Managed - I/P Only	20%
45 IP Days, 45 IP Visits, 30 OP Visits	National Avg. - 20%	$0 per Admit, $10 per OP Visit	Loosely Managed (Unmanaged)	40%
15 IP Days, 15 IP Visits, 45 OP Visits	National Avg. + 20%	$200 per Admit, $25 per OP Visit	Aggressively Managed - I/P Only	30%
30 IP Days, 30 IP Visits, 20 OP Visits	National Avg. + 20%	$0 per Admit, $10 per OP Visit	Moderately Managed - I/P & O/P	40%
45 IP Days, 45 IP Visits, 30 OP Visits	National Avg. + 20%	$0 per Admit, $10 per OP Visit	Aggressively Managed - I/P Only	40%
15 IP Days, 15 IP Visits, 45 OP Visits	National Avg. - 20%	$0 per Admit, $10 per OP Visit	Aggressively Managed - I/P Only	20%
45 IP Days, 45 IP Visits, 30 OP Visits	National Avg. - 20%	$0 per Admit, $10 per OP Visit	Moderately Managed - I/P Only	30%
15 IP Days, 15 IP Visits, 45 OP Visits	National Avg.	$200 per Admit, $25 per OP Visit	Aggressively Managed - I/P Only	20%
30 IP Days, 30 IP Visits, 20 OP Visits	National Avg.	$200 per Admit, $25 per OP Visit	Moderately Managed - I/P & O/P	20%
15 IP Days, 15 IP Visits, 45 OP Visits	National Avg. - 20%	$0 per Admit, $10 per OP Visit	Loosely Managed (Unmanaged)	30%
30 IP Days, 30 IP Visits, 20 OP Visits	National Avg. + 20%	$200 per Admit, $25 per OP Visit	Moderately Managed - I/P Only	40%
15 IP Days, 15 IP Visits, 45 OP Visits	National Avg. - 20%	$200 per Admit, $25 per OP Visit	Loosely Managed (Unmanaged)	20%
45 IP Days, 45 IP Visits, 30 OP Visits	National Avg. - 20%	$0 per Admit, $10 per OP Visit	Moderately Managed - I/P & O/P	20%
Unlimited IP Days, IP Visits, OP Visits	National Avg.	$0 per Admit, $10 per OP Visit	Aggressively Managed - I/P Only	40%
45 IP Days, 45 IP Visits, 30 OP Visits	National Avg. - 20%	$200 per Admit, $25 per OP Visit	Moderately Managed - I/P Only	20%
45 IP Days, 45 IP Visits, 30 OP Visits	National Avg.	$0 per Admit, $10 per OP Visit	Aggressively Managed - I/P Only	30%

No explicit margins or allowances for administrative expenses, coordination of benefits, stop loss reinsurance, adverse risks, or margins for profits and/or contingencies beyond those implicitly provided within the average costs per unit of service have been used.

Appendix I
Commercial Population Capitation Rates Sorted by Scenario Rate
PMPM Capitation Payments by Scenario
Estimated Psych & Substance Abuse Claim Costs as of July 1, 1995

Plan Type	Area Cost	Copay Level	Management Type	Discount Level
Capitation at least $5.50 but less than $6.00				
Unlimited IP Days, IP Visits, OP Visits	National Avg.	$200 per Admit, $25 per OP Visit	Moderately Managed - I/P & O/P	40%
45 IP Days, 45 IP Visits, 30 OP Visits	National Avg. + 20%	$200 per Admit, $25 per OP Visit	Moderately Managed - I/P & O/P	40%
30 IP Days, 30 IP Visits, 20 OP Visits	National Avg. - 20%	$200 per Admit, $25 per OP Visit	Loosely Managed (Unmanaged)	30%
15 IP Days, 15 IP Visits, 45 OP Visits	National Avg. + 20%	$200 per Admit, $25 per OP Visit	Moderately Managed - I/P & O/P	30%
30 IP Days, 30 IP Visits, 20 OP Visits	National Avg.	$0 per Admit, $10 per OP Visit	Moderately Managed - I/P & O/P	30%
15 IP Days, 15 IP Visits, 45 OP Visits	National Avg. + 20%	$0 per Admit, $10 per OP Visit	Moderately Managed - I/P & O/P	40%
30 IP Days, 30 IP Visits, 20 OP Visits	National Avg.	$200 per Admit, $25 per OP Visit	Moderately Managed - I/P Only	30%
45 IP Days, 45 IP Visits, 30 OP Visits	National Avg. + 20%	$200 per Admit, $25 per OP Visit	Aggressively Managed - I/P Only	30%
30 IP Days, 30 IP Visits, 20 OP Visits	National Avg.	$0 per Admit, $10 per OP Visit	Moderately Managed - I/P Only	40%
Unlimited IP Days, IP Visits, OP Visits	National Avg. - 20%	$0 per Admit, $10 per OP Visit	Aggressively Managed - I/P Only	30%
15 IP Days, 15 IP Visits, 45 OP Visits	National Avg.	$0 per Admit, $10 per OP Visit	Moderately Managed - I/P Only	40%
45 IP Days, 45 IP Visits, 30 OP Visits	National Avg. - 20%	$0 per Admit, $10 per OP Visit	Aggressively Managed - I/P Only	20%
45 IP Days, 45 IP Visits, 30 OP Visits	National Avg.	$200 per Admit, $25 per OP Visit	Moderately Managed - I/P & O/P	30%
30 IP Days, 30 IP Visits, 20 OP Visits	National Avg. - 20%	$0 per Admit, $10 per OP Visit	Loosely Managed (Unmanaged)	40%
45 IP Days, 45 IP Visits, 30 OP Visits	National Avg.	$200 per Admit, $25 per OP Visit	Aggressively Managed - I/P Only	20%
15 IP Days, 15 IP Visits, 45 OP Visits	National Avg. + 20%	$200 per Admit, $25 per OP Visit	Moderately Managed - I/P Only	40%
Unlimited IP Days, IP Visits, OP Visits	National Avg. + 20%	$200 per Admit, $25 per OP Visit	Aggressively Managed - I/P Only	40%
Unlimited IP Days, IP Visits, OP Visits	National Avg.	$200 per Admit, $25 per OP Visit	Aggressively Managed - I/P Only	30%
15 IP Days, 15 IP Visits, 45 OP Visits	National Avg.	$0 per Admit, $10 per OP Visit	Moderately Managed - I/P & O/P	30%
15 IP Days, 15 IP Visits, 45 OP Visits	National Avg. + 20%	$0 per Admit, $10 per OP Visit	Aggressively Managed - I/P & O/P	20%
Unlimited IP Days, IP Visits, OP Visits	National Avg. - 20%	$200 per Admit, $25 per OP Visit	Moderately Managed - I/P & O/P	30%
15 IP Days, 15 IP Visits, 45 OP Visits	National Avg.	$200 per Admit, $25 per OP Visit	Moderately Managed - I/P & O/P	20%
45 IP Days, 45 IP Visits, 30 OP Visits	National Avg.	$0 per Admit, $10 per OP Visit	Moderately Managed - I/P & O/P	40%
15 IP Days, 15 IP Visits, 45 OP Visits	National Avg.	$200 per Admit, $25 per OP Visit	Moderately Managed - I/P Only	30%
Unlimited IP Days, IP Visits, OP Visits	National Avg. - 20%	$0 per Admit, $10 per OP Visit	Moderately Managed - I/P & O/P	40%
30 IP Days, 30 IP Visits, 20 OP Visits	National Avg. + 20%	$0 per Admit, $10 per OP Visit	Aggressively Managed - I/P Only	40%

No explicit margins or allowances for administrative expenses, coordination of benefits, stop loss reinsurance, adverse risks, or margins for profits and/or contingencies beyond those implicitly provided within the average costs per unit of service have been used.

Appendix I
Commercial Population Capitation Rates Sorted by Scenario Rate
PMPM Capitation Payments by Scenario
Estimated Psych & Substance Abuse Claim Costs as of July 1, 1995

Plan Type	Area Cost	Copay Level	Management Type	Discount Level
Capitation at least $5.00 but less than $5.50				
Unlimited IP Days, IP Visits, OP Visits	National Avg. + 20%	$0 per Admit, $10 per OP Visit	Aggressively Managed - I/P & O/P	30%
30 IP Days, 30 IP Visits, 20 OP Visits	National Avg. - 20%	$0 per Admit, $10 per OP Visit	Moderately Managed - I/P Only	30%
15 IP Days, 15 IP Visits, 45 OP Visits	National Avg. - 20%	$0 per Admit, $10 per OP Visit	Moderately Managed - I/P Only	30%
Unlimited IP Days, IP Visits, OP Visits	National Avg. + 20%	$200 per Admit, $25 per OP Visit	Aggressively Managed - I/P & O/P	20%
15 IP Days, 15 IP Visits, 45 OP Visits	National Avg.	$0 per Admit, $10 per OP Visit	Aggressively Managed - I/P Only	40%
30 IP Days, 30 IP Visits, 20 OP Visits	National Avg. - 20%	$0 per Admit, $10 per OP Visit	Moderately Managed - I/P & O/P	20%
45 IP Days, 45 IP Visits, 30 OP Visits	National Avg. - 20%	$200 per Admit, $25 per OP Visit	Loosely Managed (Unmanaged)	40%
30 IP Days, 30 IP Visits, 20 OP Visits	National Avg. - 20%	$200 per Admit, $25 per OP Visit	Moderately Managed - I/P Only	20%
15 IP Days, 15 IP Visits, 45 OP Visits	National Avg.	$200 per Admit, $25 per OP Visit	Loosely Managed (Unmanaged)	40%
30 IP Days, 30 IP Visits, 20 OP Visits	National Avg. + 20%	$200 per Admit, $25 per OP Visit	Moderately Managed - I/P & O/P	40%
15 IP Days, 15 IP Visits, 45 OP Visits	National Avg. - 20%	$0 per Admit, $10 per OP Visit	Aggressively Managed - I/P Only	30%
30 IP Days, 30 IP Visits, 20 OP Visits	National Avg.	$0 per Admit, $10 per OP Visit	Aggressively Managed - I/P Only	30%
45 IP Days, 45 IP Visits, 30 OP Visits	National Avg.	$200 per Admit, $25 per OP Visit	Moderately Managed - I/P Only	40%
Unlimited IP Days, IP Visits, OP Visits	National Avg. - 20%	$200 per Admit, $25 per OP Visit	Aggressively Managed - I/P Only	20%
45 IP Days, 45 IP Visits, 30 OP Visits	National Avg. + 20%	$0 per Admit, $10 per OP Visit	Aggressively Managed - I/P & O/P	20%
45 IP Days, 45 IP Visits, 30 OP Visits	National Avg. - 20%	$200 per Admit, $25 per OP Visit	Moderately Managed - I/P & O/P	20%
45 IP Days, 45 IP Visits, 30 OP Visits	National Avg. - 20%	$0 per Admit, $10 per OP Visit	Moderately Managed - I/P & O/P	30%
30 IP Days, 30 IP Visits, 20 OP Visits	National Avg. + 20%	$200 per Admit, $25 per OP Visit	Aggressively Managed - I/P Only	30%
Unlimited IP Days, IP Visits, OP Visits	National Avg.	$0 per Admit, $10 per OP Visit	Aggressively Managed - I/P & O/P	20%
15 IP Days, 15 IP Visits, 45 OP Visits	National Avg. - 20%	$0 per Admit, $10 per OP Visit	Moderately Managed - I/P & O/P	20%
15 IP Days, 15 IP Visits, 45 OP Visits	National Avg. - 20%	$200 per Admit, $25 per OP Visit	Moderately Managed - I/P Only	20%
30 IP Days, 30 IP Visits, 20 OP Visits	National Avg.	$200 per Admit, $25 per OP Visit	Moderately Managed - I/P & O/P	30%
45 IP Days, 45 IP Visits, 30 OP Visits	National Avg. - 20%	$0 per Admit, $10 per OP Visit	Moderately Managed - I/P Only	40%
Unlimited IP Days, IP Visits, OP Visits	National Avg. - 20%	$200 per Admit, $25 per OP Visit	Moderately Managed - I/P Only	40%
15 IP Days, 15 IP Visits, 45 OP Visits	National Avg. - 20%	$0 per Admit, $10 per OP Visit	Loosely Managed (Unmanaged)	40%
30 IP Days, 30 IP Visits, 20 OP Visits	National Avg. - 20%	$0 per Admit, $10 per OP Visit	Aggressively Managed - I/P Only	20%
30 IP Days, 30 IP Visits, 20 OP Visits	National Avg.	$200 per Admit, $25 per OP Visit	Aggressively Managed - I/P Only	20%
15 IP Days, 15 IP Visits, 45 OP Visits	National Avg. - 20%	$200 per Admit, $25 per OP Visit	Loosely Managed (Unmanaged)	30%
45 IP Days, 45 IP Visits, 30 OP Visits	National Avg. - 20%	$200 per Admit, $25 per OP Visit	Moderately Managed - I/P Only	30%
45 IP Days, 45 IP Visits, 30 OP Visits	National Avg.	$0 per Admit, $10 per OP Visit	Aggressively Managed - I/P Only	40%
30 IP Days, 30 IP Visits, 20 OP Visits	National Avg.	$0 per Admit, $10 per OP Visit	Moderately Managed - I/P & O/P	40%
15 IP Days, 15 IP Visits, 45 OP Visits	National Avg.	$200 per Admit, $25 per OP Visit	Aggressively Managed - I/P Only	30%

No explicit margins or allowances for administrative expenses, coordination of benefits, stop loss reinsurance, adverse risks, or margins for profits and/or contingencies beyond those implicitly provided within the average costs per unit of service have been used.

Appendix I
Commercial Population Capitation Rates Sorted by Scenario Rate
PMPM Capitation Payments by Scenario
Estimated Psych & Substance Abuse Claim Costs as of July 1, 1995

Plan Type	Area Cost	Copay Level	Management Type	Discount Level
Capitation at least $4.50 but less than $5.00				
15 IP Days, 15 IP Visits, 45 OP Visits	National Avg. + 20%	$200 per Admit, $25 per OP Visit	Aggressively Managed - I/P Only	40%
30 IP Days, 30 IP Visits, 20 OP Visits	National Avg. - 20%	$200 per Admit, $25 per OP Visit	Loosely Managed (Unmanaged)	40%
45 IP Days, 45 IP Visits, 30 OP Visits	National Avg. - 20%	$0 per Admit, $10 per OP Visit	Aggressively Managed - I/P Only	30%
Unlimited IP Days, IP Visits, OP Visits	National Avg. - 20%	$0 per Admit, $10 per OP Visit	Aggressively Managed - I/P Only	40%
30 IP Days, 30 IP Visits, 20 OP Visits	National Avg. - 20%	$200 per Admit, $25 per OP Visit	Moderately Managed - I/P & O/P	20%
15 IP Days, 15 IP Visits, 45 OP Visits	National Avg. - 20%	$200 per Admit, $25 per OP Visit	Aggressively Managed - I/P Only	20%
15 IP Days, 15 IP Visits, 45 OP Visits	National Avg. + 20%	$200 per Admit, $25 per OP Visit	Moderately Managed - I/P & O/P	40%
30 IP Days, 30 IP Visits, 20 OP Visits	National Avg.	$200 per Admit, $25 per OP Visit	Moderately Managed - I/P Only	40%
30 IP Days, 30 IP Visits, 20 OP Visits	National Avg. + 20%	$0 per Admit, $10 per OP Visit	Aggressively Managed - I/P & O/P	20%
15 IP Days, 15 IP Visits, 45 OP Visits	National Avg. + 20%	$0 per Admit, $10 per OP Visit	Aggressively Managed - I/P & O/P	30%
15 IP Days, 15 IP Visits, 45 OP Visits	National Avg.	$0 per Admit, $10 per OP Visit	Moderately Managed - I/P & O/P	40%
45 IP Days, 45 IP Visits, 30 OP Visits	National Avg.	$200 per Admit, $25 per OP Visit	Moderately Managed - I/P & O/P	40%
30 IP Days, 30 IP Visits, 20 OP Visits	National Avg. - 20%	$0 per Admit, $10 per OP Visit	Moderately Managed - I/P & O/P	30%
15 IP Days, 15 IP Visits, 45 OP Visits	National Avg.	$200 per Admit, $25 per OP Visit	Moderately Managed - I/P & O/P	30%
15 IP Days, 15 IP Visits, 45 OP Visits	National Avg. + 20%	$200 per Admit, $25 per OP Visit	Aggressively Managed - I/P & O/P	20%
45 IP Days, 45 IP Visits, 30 OP Visits	National Avg.	$200 per Admit, $25 per OP Visit	Aggressively Managed - I/P Only	30%
45 IP Days, 45 IP Visits, 30 OP Visits	National Avg. + 20%	$200 per Admit, $25 per OP Visit	Aggressively Managed - I/P Only	40%
Unlimited IP Days, IP Visits, OP Visits	National Avg. + 20%	$0 per Admit, $10 per OP Visit	Aggressively Managed - I/P & O/P	40%
30 IP Days, 30 IP Visits, 20 OP Visits	National Avg. - 20%	$0 per Admit, $10 per OP Visit	Moderately Managed - I/P Only	40%
Unlimited IP Days, IP Visits, OP Visits	National Avg. - 20%	$200 per Admit, $25 per OP Visit	Moderately Managed - I/P & O/P	40%
15 IP Days, 15 IP Visits, 45 OP Visits	National Avg. - 20%	$0 per Admit, $10 per OP Visit	Moderately Managed - I/P Only	40%
15 IP Days, 15 IP Visits, 45 OP Visits	National Avg.	$0 per Admit, $10 per OP Visit	Aggressively Managed - I/P & O/P	20%
Unlimited IP Days, IP Visits, OP Visits	National Avg. + 20%	$200 per Admit, $25 per OP Visit	Aggressively Managed - I/P & O/P	30%
30 IP Days, 30 IP Visits, 20 OP Visits	National Avg. - 20%	$200 per Admit, $25 per OP Visit	Moderately Managed - I/P Only	30%
30 IP Days, 30 IP Visits, 20 OP Visits	National Avg.	$0 per Admit, $10 per OP Visit	Aggressively Managed - I/P Only	40%
45 IP Days, 45 IP Visits, 30 OP Visits	National Avg. - 20%	$200 per Admit, $25 per OP Visit	Aggressively Managed - I/P Only	20%
15 IP Days, 15 IP Visits, 45 OP Visits	National Avg.	$200 per Admit, $25 per OP Visit	Moderately Managed - I/P Only	40%
15 IP Days, 15 IP Visits, 45 OP Visits	National Avg. - 20%	$0 per Admit, $10 per OP Visit	Moderately Managed - I/P & O/P	30%

No explicit margins or allowances for administrative expenses, coordination of benefits, stop loss reinsurance, adverse risks, or margins for profits and/or contingencies beyond those implicitly provided within the average costs per unit of service have been used.

Appendix I
Commercial Population Capitation Rates Sorted by Scenario Rate
PMPM Capitation Payments by Scenario
Estimated Psych & Substance Abuse Claim Costs as of July 1, 1995

Plan Type	Area Cost	Copay Level	Management Type	Discount Level
Capitation at least $4.00 but less than $4.50				
15 IP Days, 15 IP Visits, 45 OP Visits	National Avg. - 20%	$0 per Admit, $10 per OP Visit	Aggressively Managed - I/P Only	40%
45 IP Days, 45 IP Visits, 30 OP Visits	National Avg. + 20%	$0 per Admit, $10 per OP Visit	Aggressively Managed - I/P & O/P	30%
Unlimited IP Days, IP Visits, OP Visits	National Avg.	$200 per Admit, $25 per OP Visit	Aggressively Managed - I/P Only	40%
45 IP Days, 45 IP Visits, 30 OP Visits	National Avg. - 20%	$200 per Admit, $25 per OP Visit	Moderately Managed - I/P & O/P	30%
45 IP Days, 45 IP Visits, 30 OP Visits	National Avg. - 20%	$0 per Admit, $10 per OP Visit	Moderately Managed - I/P & O/P	40%
Unlimited IP Days, IP Visits, OP Visits	National Avg.	$0 per Admit, $10 per OP Visit	Aggressively Managed - I/P & O/P	30%
45 IP Days, 45 IP Visits, 30 OP Visits	National Avg. + 20%	$200 per Admit, $25 per OP Visit	Aggressively Managed - I/P & O/P	20%
30 IP Days, 30 IP Visits, 20 OP Visits	National Avg. - 20%	$0 per Admit, $10 per OP Visit	Aggressively Managed - I/P Only	30%
Unlimited IP Days, IP Visits, OP Visits	National Avg.	$200 per Admit, $25 per OP Visit	Aggressively Managed - I/P & O/P	20%
15 IP Days, 15 IP Visits, 45 OP Visits	National Avg. - 20%	$200 per Admit, $25 per OP Visit	Moderately Managed - I/P & O/P	20%
Unlimited IP Days, IP Visits, OP Visits	National Avg. - 20%	$200 per Admit, $25 per OP Visit	Aggressively Managed - I/P Only	30%
45 IP Days, 45 IP Visits, 30 OP Visits	National Avg.	$0 per Admit, $10 per OP Visit	Aggressively Managed - I/P & O/P	20%
15 IP Days, 15 IP Visits, 45 OP Visits	National Avg. - 20%	$200 per Admit, $25 per OP Visit	Moderately Managed - I/P Only	30%
30 IP Days, 30 IP Visits, 20 OP Visits	National Avg.	$200 per Admit, $25 per OP Visit	Moderately Managed - I/P & O/P	40%
30 IP Days, 30 IP Visits, 20 OP Visits	National Avg.	$200 per Admit, $25 per OP Visit	Aggressively Managed - I/P Only	30%
30 IP Days, 30 IP Visits, 20 OP Visits	National Avg. + 20%	$200 per Admit, $25 per OP Visit	Aggressively Managed - I/P Only	40%
30 IP Days, 30 IP Visits, 20 OP Visits	National Avg. - 20%	$200 per Admit, $25 per OP Visit	Moderately Managed - I/P & O/P	30%
15 IP Days, 15 IP Visits, 45 OP Visits	National Avg. - 20%	$200 per Admit, $25 per OP Visit	Loosely Managed (Unmanaged)	40%
45 IP Days, 45 IP Visits, 30 OP Visits	National Avg. - 20%	$0 per Admit, $10 per OP Visit	Aggressively Managed - I/P Only	40%
Unlimited IP Days, IP Visits, OP Visits	National Avg. - 20%	$0 per Admit, $10 per OP Visit	Aggressively Managed - I/P & O/P	20%
45 IP Days, 45 IP Visits, 30 OP Visits	National Avg. - 20%	$200 per Admit, $25 per OP Visit	Moderately Managed - I/P Only	40%
30 IP Days, 30 IP Visits, 20 OP Visits	National Avg. + 20%	$0 per Admit, $10 per OP Visit	Aggressively Managed - I/P & O/P	30%
30 IP Days, 30 IP Visits, 20 OP Visits	National Avg. + 20%	$200 per Admit, $25 per OP Visit	Aggressively Managed - I/P & O/P	20%
30 IP Days, 30 IP Visits, 20 OP Visits	National Avg. - 20%	$200 per Admit, $25 per OP Visit	Aggressively Managed - I/P Only	20%
15 IP Days, 15 IP Visits, 45 OP Visits	National Avg. + 20%	$0 per Admit, $10 per OP Visit	Aggressively Managed - I/P & O/P	40%

No explicit margins or allowances for administrative expenses, coordination of benefits, stop loss reinsurance, adverse risks, or margins for profits and/or contingencies beyond those implicitly provided within the average costs per unit of service have been used.

Appendix I
Commercial Population Capitation Rates Sorted by Scenario Rate
PMPM Capitation Payments by Scenario
Estimated Psych & Substance Abuse Claim Costs as of July 1, 1995

Plan Type	Area Cost	Copay Level	Management Type	Discount Level
Capitation at least $3.50 but less than $4.00				
30 IP Days, 30 IP Visits, 20 OP Visits	National Avg. - 20%	$0 per Admit, $10 per OP Visit	Moderately Managed - I/P & O/P	40%
15 IP Days, 15 IP Visits, 45 OP Visits	National Avg.	$200 per Admit, $25 per OP Visit	Aggressively Managed - I/P Only	40%
30 IP Days, 30 IP Visits, 20 OP Visits	National Avg.	$0 per Admit, $10 per OP Visit	Aggressively Managed - I/P & O/P	20%
15 IP Days, 15 IP Visits, 45 OP Visits	National Avg. - 20%	$200 per Admit, $25 per OP Visit	Aggressively Managed - I/P Only	30%
15 IP Days, 15 IP Visits, 45 OP Visits	National Avg.	$0 per Admit, $10 per OP Visit	Aggressively Managed - I/P & O/P	30%
15 IP Days, 15 IP Visits, 45 OP Visits	National Avg. + 20%	$200 per Admit, $25 per OP Visit	Aggressively Managed - I/P & O/P	30%
15 IP Days, 15 IP Visits, 45 OP Visits	National Avg.	$200 per Admit, $25 per OP Visit	Moderately Managed - I/P & O/P	40%
15 IP Days, 15 IP Visits, 45 OP Visits	National Avg. - 20%	$0 per Admit, $10 per OP Visit	Moderately Managed - I/P & O/P	40%
15 IP Days, 15 IP Visits, 45 OP Visits	National Avg.	$200 per Admit, $25 per OP Visit	Aggressively Managed - I/P & O/P	20%
45 IP Days, 45 IP Visits, 30 OP Visits	National Avg. + 20%	$0 per Admit, $10 per OP Visit	Aggressively Managed - I/P & O/P	40%
Unlimited IP Days, IP Visits, OP Visits	National Avg.	$0 per Admit, $10 per OP Visit	Aggressively Managed - I/P & O/P	40%
15 IP Days, 15 IP Visits, 45 OP Visits	National Avg. - 20%	$0 per Admit, $10 per OP Visit	Aggressively Managed - I/P & O/P	20%
Unlimited IP Days, IP Visits, OP Visits	National Avg. + 20%	$200 per Admit, $25 per OP Visit	Aggressively Managed - I/P & O/P	40%
30 IP Days, 30 IP Visits, 20 OP Visits	National Avg. - 20%	$0 per Admit, $10 per OP Visit	Aggressively Managed - I/P Only	40%
45 IP Days, 45 IP Visits, 30 OP Visits	National Avg.	$200 per Admit, $25 per OP Visit	Aggressively Managed - I/P Only	40%
30 IP Days, 30 IP Visits, 20 OP Visits	National Avg. - 20%	$200 per Admit, $25 per OP Visit	Moderately Managed - I/P Only	40%
45 IP Days, 45 IP Visits, 30 OP Visits	National Avg. - 20%	$200 per Admit, $25 per OP Visit	Aggressively Managed - I/P Only	30%
45 IP Days, 45 IP Visits, 30 OP Visits	National Avg. + 20%	$200 per Admit, $25 per OP Visit	Aggressively Managed - I/P & O/P	30%
45 IP Days, 45 IP Visits, 30 OP Visits	National Avg.	$0 per Admit, $10 per OP Visit	Aggressively Managed - I/P & O/P	30%
45 IP Days, 45 IP Visits, 30 OP Visits	National Avg. - 20%	$200 per Admit, $25 per OP Visit	Moderately Managed - I/P & O/P	40%
Unlimited IP Days, IP Visits, OP Visits	National Avg.	$200 per Admit, $25 per OP Visit	Aggressively Managed - I/P & O/P	30%
15 IP Days, 15 IP Visits, 45 OP Visits	National Avg. - 20%	$200 per Admit, $25 per OP Visit	Moderately Managed - I/P & O/P	30%
45 IP Days, 45 IP Visits, 30 OP Visits	National Avg.	$200 per Admit, $25 per OP Visit	Aggressively Managed - I/P & O/P	20%
Unlimited IP Days, IP Visits, OP Visits	National Avg. - 20%	$0 per Admit, $10 per OP Visit	Aggressively Managed - I/P & O/P	30%
45 IP Days, 45 IP Visits, 30 OP Visits	National Avg. - 20%	$0 per Admit, $10 per OP Visit	Aggressively Managed - I/P & O/P	20%
30 IP Days, 30 IP Visits, 20 OP Visits	National Avg. - 20%	$0 per Admit, $10 per OP Visit	Aggressively Managed - I/P & O/P	20%
30 IP Days, 30 IP Visits, 20 OP Visits	National Avg.	$200 per Admit, $25 per OP Visit	Aggressively Managed - I/P & O/P	20%

No explicit margins or allowances for administrative expenses, coordination of benefits, stop loss reinsurance, adverse risks, or margins for profits and/or contingencies beyond those implicitly provided within the average costs per unit of service have been used.

Appendix I
Commercial Population Capitation Rates Sorted by Scenario Rate
PMPM Capitation Payments by Scenario
Estimated Psych & Substance Abuse Claim Costs as of July 1, 1995

Plan Type	Area Cost	Copay Level	Management Type	Discount Level
Capitation at least $3.00 but less than $3.50				
30 IP Days, 30 IP Visits, 20 OP Visits	National Avg. + 20%	$200 per Admit, $25 per OP Visit	Aggressively Managed - I/P & O/P	30%
15 IP Days, 15 IP Visits, 45 OP Visits	National Avg. - 20%	$200 per Admit, $25 per OP Visit	Moderately Managed - I/P Only	40%
30 IP Days, 30 IP Visits, 20 OP Visits	National Avg. - 20%	$200 per Admit, $25 per OP Visit	Moderately Managed - I/P & O/P	40%
30 IP Days, 30 IP Visits, 20 OP Visits	National Avg. + 20%	$0 per Admit, $10 per OP Visit	Aggressively Managed - I/P & O/P	40%
30 IP Days, 30 IP Visits, 20 OP Visits	National Avg.	$0 per Admit, $10 per OP Visit	Aggressively Managed - I/P & O/P	30%
Unlimited IP Days, IP Visits, OP Visits	National Avg. - 20%	$200 per Admit, $25 per OP Visit	Aggressively Managed - I/P Only	40%
Unlimited IP Days, IP Visits, OP Visits	National Avg. - 20%	$200 per Admit, $25 per OP Visit	Aggressively Managed - I/P & O/P	20%
30 IP Days, 30 IP Visits, 20 OP Visits	National Avg.	$200 per Admit, $25 per OP Visit	Aggressively Managed - I/P Only	40%
30 IP Days, 30 IP Visits, 20 OP Visits	National Avg. - 20%	$200 per Admit, $25 per OP Visit	Aggressively Managed - I/P Only	30%
15 IP Days, 15 IP Visits, 45 OP Visits	National Avg.	$0 per Admit, $10 per OP Visit	Aggressively Managed - I/P & O/P	40%
15 IP Days, 15 IP Visits, 45 OP Visits	National Avg. - 20%	$0 per Admit, $10 per OP Visit	Aggressively Managed - I/P & O/P	30%
15 IP Days, 15 IP Visits, 45 OP Visits	National Avg. + 20%	$200 per Admit, $25 per OP Visit	Aggressively Managed - I/P & O/P	40%
15 IP Days, 15 IP Visits, 45 OP Visits	National Avg.	$200 per Admit, $25 per OP Visit	Aggressively Managed - I/P & O/P	30%
15 IP Days, 15 IP Visits, 45 OP Visits	National Avg. - 20%	$200 per Admit, $25 per OP Visit	Aggressively Managed - I/P Only	40%
45 IP Days, 45 IP Visits, 30 OP Visits	National Avg.	$0 per Admit, $10 per OP Visit	Aggressively Managed - I/P & O/P	40%
30 IP Days, 30 IP Visits, 20 OP Visits	National Avg. - 20%	$0 per Admit, $10 per OP Visit	Aggressively Managed - I/P & O/P	30%
45 IP Days, 45 IP Visits, 30 OP Visits	National Avg. - 20%	$0 per Admit, $10 per OP Visit	Aggressively Managed - I/P & O/P	30%
45 IP Days, 45 IP Visits, 30 OP Visits	National Avg. - 20%	$200 per Admit, $25 per OP Visit	Aggressively Managed - I/P & O/P	20%
15 IP Days, 15 IP Visits, 45 OP Visits	National Avg. - 20%	$200 per Admit, $25 per OP Visit	Aggressively Managed - I/P & O/P	20%
30 IP Days, 30 IP Visits, 20 OP Visits	National Avg. - 20%	$200 per Admit, $25 per OP Visit	Aggressively Managed - I/P & O/P	20%
Unlimited IP Days, IP Visits, OP Visits	National Avg. - 20%	$0 per Admit, $10 per OP Visit	Aggressively Managed - I/P & O/P	40%
Capitation at least $2.50 but less than $3.00				
45 IP Days, 45 IP Visits, 30 OP Visits	National Avg. + 20%	$200 per Admit, $25 per OP Visit	Aggressively Managed - I/P & O/P	40%
45 IP Days, 45 IP Visits, 30 OP Visits	National Avg.	$200 per Admit, $25 per OP Visit	Aggressively Managed - I/P & O/P	30%
30 IP Days, 30 IP Visits, 20 OP Visits	National Avg.	$200 per Admit, $25 per OP Visit	Aggressively Managed - I/P & O/P	30%
15 IP Days, 15 IP Visits, 45 OP Visits	National Avg. - 20%	$200 per Admit, $25 per OP Visit	Moderately Managed - I/P & O/P	40%
Unlimited IP Days, IP Visits, OP Visits	National Avg.	$200 per Admit, $25 per OP Visit	Aggressively Managed - I/P & O/P	40%
45 IP Days, 45 IP Visits, 30 OP Visits	National Avg. - 20%	$200 per Admit, $25 per OP Visit	Aggressively Managed - I/P Only	40%
30 IP Days, 30 IP Visits, 20 OP Visits	National Avg.	$0 per Admit, $10 per OP Visit	Aggressively Managed - I/P & O/P	40%
30 IP Days, 30 IP Visits, 20 OP Visits	National Avg. + 20%	$200 per Admit, $25 per OP Visit	Aggressively Managed - I/P & O/P	40%
Unlimited IP Days, IP Visits, OP Visits	National Avg. - 20%	$200 per Admit, $25 per OP Visit	Aggressively Managed - I/P & O/P	30%
15 IP Days, 15 IP Visits, 45 OP Visits	National Avg. - 20%	$0 per Admit, $10 per OP Visit	Aggressively Managed - I/P & O/P	40%
30 IP Days, 30 IP Visits, 20 OP Visits	National Avg. - 20%	$200 per Admit, $25 per OP Visit	Aggressively Managed - I/P Only	40%
30 IP Days, 30 IP Visits, 20 OP Visits	National Avg. - 20%	$200 per Admit, $25 per OP Visit	Aggressively Managed - I/P & O/P	30%
45 IP Days, 45 IP Visits, 30 OP Visits	National Avg. - 20%	$200 per Admit, $25 per OP Visit	Aggressively Managed - I/P & O/P	30%
15 IP Days, 15 IP Visits, 45 OP Visits	National Avg. - 20%	$200 per Admit, $25 per OP Visit	Aggressively Managed - I/P & O/P	30%
30 IP Days, 30 IP Visits, 20 OP Visits	National Avg. - 20%	$0 per Admit, $10 per OP Visit	Aggressively Managed - I/P & O/P	40%
45 IP Days, 45 IP Visits, 30 OP Visits	National Avg. - 20%	$0 per Admit, $10 per OP Visit	Aggressively Managed - I/P & O/P	40%
15 IP Days, 15 IP Visits, 45 OP Visits	National Avg.	$200 per Admit, $25 per OP Visit	Aggressively Managed - I/P & O/P	40%
Capitation at least $2.00 but less than $2.50				
30 IP Days, 30 IP Visits, 20 OP Visits	National Avg.	$200 per Admit, $25 per OP Visit	Aggressively Managed - I/P & O/P	40%
45 IP Days, 45 IP Visits, 30 OP Visits	National Avg.	$200 per Admit, $25 per OP Visit	Aggressively Managed - I/P & O/P	40%
Unlimited IP Days, IP Visits, OP Visits	National Avg. - 20%	$200 per Admit, $25 per OP Visit	Aggressively Managed - I/P & O/P	40%
15 IP Days, 15 IP Visits, 45 OP Visits	National Avg. - 20%	$200 per Admit, $25 per OP Visit	Aggressively Managed - I/P & O/P	40%
45 IP Days, 45 IP Visits, 30 OP Visits	National Avg. - 20%	$200 per Admit, $25 per OP Visit	Aggressively Managed - I/P & O/P	40%
30 IP Days, 30 IP Visits, 20 OP Visits	National Avg. - 20%	$200 per Admit, $25 per OP Visit	Aggressively Managed - I/P & O/P	40%

No explicit margins or allowances for administrative expenses, coordination of benefits, stop loss reinsurance, adverse risks, or margins for profits and/or contingencies beyond those implicitly provided within the average costs per unit of service have been used.

APPENDIX II

DEVELOPMENT OF ASSUMPTIONS, MEDICARE AND MEDICAID POPULATIONS

Medicare Population

There are many variables applicable to the Medicare population that can contribute to variations in behavioral healthcare utilization and costs, including

◆ Demographics of Medicare eligible population
◆ Geographic area variations
◆ Continuum of behavioral healthcare services available
◆ Composition of professional providers by service area

Additionally, there is considerable variation in average costs per unit of service due to geographic cost differences, the types and mix of services and facilities available (e.g., acute inpatient, residential, intensive non-residential, etc.), and the types of professionals providing behavioral services to seniors (e.g., psychiatrist, psychologist, LCSW, etc.)

In order to develop utilization and cost scenarios which we considered to be representative of high, mid, and low levels across various Medicare population groups and varying levels of managed care delivery, we analyzed the following sources of behavioral healthcare utilization and cost information:

◆ M&R Health Cost Guidelines—Ages 65 and Over
◆ M&R Healthcare Management Guidelines—Medicare Population
◆ HCFA BMAD files—Physician Utilization and Cost Components

The M&R Health Cost Guidelines contain utilization and average unit cost information for behavioral healthcare benefits provided through traditional, undiscounted Medicare-allowable cost environments and for alternative delivery systems which incorporate managed care principles and modified reimbursement methods, such as HMOs, PPOs and PHOs. These Guidelines include area variations in utilization, average charges and claim costs by state and/or MSA. These variations were used to set the national, high and low utilization and average unit cost scenarios in the various capitation rate calculations.

The M&R Healthcare Management Guidelines contain utilization variations for various levels of managed care delivery, reflecting differing degrees of use of inpatient care protocols for the "uncomplicated patient," incorporating concepts of medically necessary care delivery.

The HCFA BMAD files contain actual utilization, allowed charges and billed charges based on various defining parameters. Extracts were developed from these files to develop physician service utilization and average allowed charge differences by state. These variations were used to develop the national, high and low utilization and average unit cost scenarios for professional services in the various capitation rate calculations.

Medicaid Population

There are many variables applicable to the Medicaid population that contribute to the potential for wide variation in behavioral healthcare utilization, including

♦ Composition of Medicaid eligible groups
♦ Demographics of Medicaid eligible population
♦ Geographic area variations
♦ Continuum of behavioral healthcare services available
♦ Composition of professional providers by service area

Additionally, there is considerable variation in average costs per unit of service due to geographic cost differences, the types and mix of services and facilities available (e.g., acute inpatient, residential, intensive non-residential, etc.), and the types of professionals providing behavioral services (e.g., psychiatrist, psychologist, LCSW, etc.).

In order to develop utilization and cost scenarios which we considered to be representative of high, mid, and low levels across various Medicaid population groups and varying levels of managed care delivery, we analyzed the following available sources of behavioral healthcare utilization and expenditure information:

♦ National Association of State Mental Health Program Directors (NASMHPD) Survey of 1993 Medicaid-specific Expenditures and Eligibles (22 states contributed)
♦ Behavioral healthcare cost and utilization projections by state and Medicaid eligibility category for Colorado, Iowa, Massachusetts and Tennessee
♦ Managed behavioral healthcare projections of M&R
♦ Published AMBHA managed Medicaid experience (predominantly AFDC)

We selected composite facility and professional utilization levels, average unit costs per facility day and per professional visit, and per member per month case management costs to be representative of high, mid, and low levels of utilization and costs observed in our analyses, incorporating different average risk levels of the underlying population and level of care management (loosely managed vs. moderately managed vs. aggressively managed delivery of behavioral healthcare).

Detailed Results for the Medicare Population, Sorted by Capitation Rate

We developed capitation rates in this report by applying actuarial relationships among benefit limits, local costs, degree of healthcare management, patient cost sharing, and provider discounts for ADM services. Certain combinations of these factors (e.g., low benefit plans combined with low local cost levels, aggressive care management, high patient cost sharing, and large provider discounts) produce low capitation rates. We recognize the APA's concerns that overly low capitation rates simply may not allow physicians to provide an adequate amount of care. Certainly, poor quality or poor access can occur in plans that appear to offer generous benefits or reimbursement. We do not intend for this report to be used by organizations to justify inadequate capitation rates for ADM providers. Rather, we present rates associated with these various combinations of factors in order to provide general guidance and education to APA members on these capitation issues.

Appendix III
Medicare Population Capitation Rates Sorted by Scenario Rate
PMPM Capitation Payments by Scenario
Estimated Psych & Substance Abuse Costs as of July 1, 1995

Utilization Level	Cost Level	Copay Level	Management Type	% of Medicare Allowable
Capitation at least $9.00 but less than $10.00				
High	High	None	Unmanaged Care	100%
High	High	$250 per I/P Admit, $5 per Visit	Unmanaged Care	100%
Capitation at least $8.00 but less than $9.00				
High	High	$500 per I/P Admit, $10 per Visit	Unmanaged Care	100%
High	High	None	Unmanaged Care	90%
High	National	None	Unmanaged Care	100%
High	High	$250 per I/P Admit, $5 per Visit	Unmanaged Care	90%
High	National	$250 per I/P Admit, $5 per Visit	Unmanaged Care	100%
Capitation at least $7.50 but less than $8.00				
High	High	$500 per I/P Admit, $10 per Visit	Unmanaged Care	90%
High	High	None	Moderately Managed Care, Inpatient Only	100%
High	National	$500 per I/P Admit, $10 per Visit	Unmanaged Care	100%
High	High	None	Unmanaged Care	80%
High	National	None	Unmanaged Care	90%
Capitation at least $7.00 but less than $7.50				
High	High	$250 per I/P Admit, $5 per Visit	Moderately Managed Care, Inpatient Only	100%
High	Low	None	Unmanaged Care	100%
High	High	$250 per I/P Admit, $5 per Visit	Unmanaged Care	80%
High	National	$250 per I/P Admit, $5 per Visit	Unmanaged Care	90%
National	High	None	Unmanaged Care	100%
High	High	$500 per I/P Admit, $10 per Visit	Moderately Managed Care, Inpatient Only	100%
High	High	None	Moderately Managed Care, Inpatient Only	90%
Capitation at least $6.50 but less than $7.00				
High	National	None	Moderately Managed Care, Inpatient Only	100%
High	High	$500 per I/P Admit, $10 per Visit	Unmanaged Care	80%
High	Low	$250 per I/P Admit, $5 per Visit	Unmanaged Care	100%
High	National	$500 per I/P Admit, $10 per Visit	Unmanaged Care	90%
National	High	$250 per I/P Admit, $5 per Visit	Unmanaged Care	100%
High	High	$250 per I/P Admit, $5 per Visit	Moderately Managed Care, Inpatient Only	90%
High	High	None	Moderately Managed Care, Inpatient and Outpatient	100%
High	National	None	Unmanaged Care	80%
High	National	$250 per I/P Admit, $5 per Visit	Moderately Managed Care, Inpatient Only	100%
High	Low	$500 per I/P Admit, $10 per Visit	Unmanaged Care	100%
High	Low	None	Unmanaged Care	90%
National	High	$500 per I/P Admit, $10 per Visit	Unmanaged Care	100%
Capitation at least $6.00 but less than $6.50				
High	High	$250 per I/P Admit, $5 per Visit	Moderately Managed Care, Inpatient and Outpatient	100%
National	High	None	Unmanaged Care	90%
High	National	$250 per I/P Admit, $5 per Visit	Unmanaged Care	80%
High	High	None	Aggressively Managed Care, Inpatient Only	100%
High	High	$500 per I/P Admit, $10 per Visit	Moderately Managed Care, Inpatient Only	90%
National	National	None	Unmanaged Care	100%
High	National	$500 per I/P Admit, $10 per Visit	Moderately Managed Care, Inpatient Only	100%
High	National	None	Moderately Managed Care, Inpatient Only	90%
High	Low	$250 per I/P Admit, $5 per Visit	Unmanaged Care	90%
High	High	None	Moderately Managed Care, Inpatient Only	80%
High	Low	None	Moderately Managed Care, Inpatient Only	100%
High	High	$500 per I/P Admit, $10 per Visit	Moderately Managed Care, Inpatient and Outpatient	100%
National	High	$250 per I/P Admit, $5 per Visit	Unmanaged Care	90%
High	National	$500 per I/P Admit, $10 per Visit	Unmanaged Care	80%
High	High	$250 per I/P Admit, $5 per Visit	Aggressively Managed Care, Inpatient Only	100%
National	National	$250 per I/P Admit, $5 per Visit	Unmanaged Care	100%
High	High	None	Moderately Managed Care, Inpatient and Outpatient	90%

No explicit margins or allowances for administrative expenses, coordination of benefits, stop loss reinsurance, adverse risks, or margins for profits and/or contingencies beyond those implicitly provided within the average costs per unit of service have been used.

Appendix III
Medicare Population Capitation Rates Sorted by Scenario Rate
PMPM Capitation Payments by Scenario
Estimated Psych & Substance Abuse Costs as of July 1, 1995

Utilization Level	Cost Level	Copay Level	Management Type	% of Medicare Allowable
Capitation at least $5.50 but less than $6.00				
High	National	$250 per I/P Admit, $5 per Visit	Moderately Managed Care, Inpatient Only	90%
High	National	None	Moderately Managed Care, Inpatient and Outpatient	100%
High	High	$250 per I/P Admit, $5 per Visit	Moderately Managed Care, Inpatient Only	80%
High	Low	$500 per I/P Admit, $10 per Visit	Unmanaged Care	90%
National	High	$500 per I/P Admit, $10 per Visit	Unmanaged Care	90%
High	Low	None	Unmanaged Care	80%
National	High	None	Moderately Managed Care, Inpatient Only	100%
High	Low	$250 per I/P Admit, $5 per Visit	Moderately Managed Care, Inpatient Only	100%
High	National	None	Aggressively Managed Care, Inpatient Only	100%
High	High	$250 per I/P Admit, $5 per Visit	Moderately Managed Care, Inpatient and Outpatient	90%
High	High	$500 per I/P Admit, $10 per Visit	Aggressively Managed Care, Inpatient Only	100%
High	High	None	Aggressively Managed Care, Inpatient Only	90%
National	National	$500 per I/P Admit, $10 per Visit	Unmanaged Care	100%
High	National	$250 per I/P Admit, $5 per Visit	Moderately Managed Care, Inpatient and Outpatient	100%
National	High	None	Unmanaged Care	80%
National	National	None	Unmanaged Care	90%
High	High	$500 per I/P Admit, $10 per Visit	Moderately Managed Care, Inpatient Only	80%
High	National	$500 per I/P Admit, $10 per Visit	Moderately Managed Care, Inpatient Only	90%
National	High	$250 per I/P Admit, $5 per Visit	Moderately Managed Care, Inpatient Only	100%
High	National	None	Moderately Managed Care, Inpatient Only	80%
High	Low	$250 per I/P Admit, $5 per Visit	Unmanaged Care	80%
High	Low	None	Moderately Managed Care, Inpatient Only	90%
High	High	$500 per I/P Admit, $10 per Visit	Moderately Managed Care, Inpatient and Outpatient	90%
National	Low	None	Unmanaged Care	100%
High	Low	$500 per I/P Admit, $10 per Visit	Moderately Managed Care, Inpatient Only	100%
High	National	$250 per I/P Admit, $5 per Visit	Aggressively Managed Care, Inpatient Only	100%
Capitation at least $5.00 but less than $5.50				
High	High	$250 per I/P Admit, $5 per Visit	Aggressively Managed Care, Inpatient Only	90%
National	High	$250 per I/P Admit, $5 per Visit	Unmanaged Care	80%
High	National	$500 per I/P Admit, $10 per Visit	Moderately Managed Care, Inpatient and Outpatient	100%
National	National	$250 per I/P Admit, $5 per Visit	Unmanaged Care	90%
High	National	None	Moderately Managed Care, Inpatient and Outpatient	90%
High	High	None	Moderately Managed Care, Inpatient and Outpatient	80%
National	High	$500 per I/P Admit, $10 per Visit	Moderately Managed Care, Inpatient Only	100%
High	National	$250 per I/P Admit, $5 per Visit	Moderately Managed Care, Inpatient Only	80%
High	Low	$500 per I/P Admit, $10 per Visit	Unmanaged Care	80%
High	Low	$250 per I/P Admit, $5 per Visit	Moderately Managed Care, Inpatient Only	90%
National	High	None	Moderately Managed Care, Inpatient Only	90%
High	National	None	Aggressively Managed Care, Inpatient Only	90%
High	Low	None	Moderately Managed Care, Inpatient and Outpatient	100%
National	High	$500 per I/P Admit, $10 per Visit	Unmanaged Care	80%
High	Low	None	Aggressively Managed Care, Inpatient Only	100%
National	National	None	Moderately Managed Care, Inpatient Only	100%
National	Low	$250 per I/P Admit, $5 per Visit	Unmanaged Care	100%
High	National	$500 per I/P Admit, $10 per Visit	Aggressively Managed Care, Inpatient Only	100%
High	High	$500 per I/P Admit, $10 per Visit	Aggressively Managed Care, Inpatient Only	90%
National	National	$500 per I/P Admit, $10 per Visit	Unmanaged Care	90%
High	High	$250 per I/P Admit, $5 per Visit	Moderately Managed Care, Inpatient and Outpatient	80%
High	National	$250 per I/P Admit, $5 per Visit	Moderately Managed Care, Inpatient and Outpatient	90%
High	High	None	Aggressively Managed Care, Inpatient Only	80%
National	National	None	Unmanaged Care	80%
High	National	$500 per I/P Admit, $10 per Visit	Moderately Managed Care, Inpatient Only	80%
National	High	None	Moderately Managed Care, Inpatient and Outpatient	100%
Low	High	None	Unmanaged Care	100%
National	High	$250 per I/P Admit, $5 per Visit	Moderately Managed Care, Inpatient Only	90%

No explicit margins or allowances for administrative expenses, coordination of benefits, stop loss reinsurance, adverse risks, or margins for profits and/or contingencies beyond those implicitly provided within the average costs per unit of service have been used.

Appendix III
Medicare Population Capitation Rates Sorted by Scenario Rate
PMPM Capitation Payments by Scenario
Estimated Psych & Substance Abuse Costs as of July 1, 1995

Utilization Level	Cost Level	Copay Level	Management Type	% of Medicare Allowable
Capitation at least $4.75 but less than $5.00				
National	National	$250 per I/P Admit, $5 per Visit	Moderately Managed Care, Inpatient Only	100%
High	Low	$250 per I/P Admit, $5 per Visit	Moderately Managed Care, Inpatient and Outpatient	100%
National	Low	None	Unmanaged Care	90%
High	Low	$500 per I/P Admit, $10 per Visit	Moderately Managed Care, Inpatient Only	90%
High	National	$250 per I/P Admit, $5 per Visit	Aggressively Managed Care, Inpatient Only	90%
High	Low	None	Moderately Managed Care, Inpatient Only	80%
National	Low	$500 per I/P Admit, $10 per Visit	Unmanaged Care	100%
High	High	$500 per I/P Admit, $10 per Visit	Moderately Managed Care, Inpatient and Outpatient	80%
High	Low	$250 per I/P Admit, $5 per Visit	Aggressively Managed Care, Inpatient Only	100%
High	National	$500 per I/P Admit, $10 per Visit	Moderately Managed Care, Inpatient and Outpatient	90%
High	High	$250 per I/P Admit, $5 per Visit	Aggressively Managed Care, Inpatient Only	80%
National	High	$250 per I/P Admit, $5 per Visit	Moderately Managed Care, Inpatient and Outpatient	100%
Low	High	$250 per I/P Admit, $5 per Visit	Unmanaged Care	100%
National	National	$250 per I/P Admit, $5 per Visit	Unmanaged Care	80%
National	High	$500 per I/P Admit, $10 per Visit	Moderately Managed Care, Inpatient Only	90%
High	National	None	Moderately Managed Care, Inpatient and Outpatient	80%
National	High	None	Aggressively Managed Care, Inpatient Only	100%
Capitation at least $4.50 but less than $4.75				
National	National	$500 per I/P Admit, $10 per Visit	Moderately Managed Care, Inpatient Only	100%
National	National	None	Moderately Managed Care, Inpatient Only	90%
High	Low	None	Aggressively Managed Care, Inpatient Only	90%
High	Low	None	Moderately Managed Care, Inpatient and Outpatient	90%
National	Low	$250 per I/P Admit, $5 per Visit	Unmanaged Care	90%
High	Low	$500 per I/P Admit, $10 per Visit	Moderately Managed Care, Inpatient and Outpatient	100%
High	Low	$250 per I/P Admit, $5 per Visit	Moderately Managed Care, Inpatient Only	80%
High	National	$500 per I/P Admit, $10 per Visit	Aggressively Managed Care, Inpatient Only	90%
National	High	None	Moderately Managed Care, Inpatient Only	80%
High	National	None	Aggressively Managed Care, Inpatient Only	80%
National	Low	None	Moderately Managed Care, Inpatient Only	100%
High	High	$500 per I/P Admit, $10 per Visit	Aggressively Managed Care, Inpatient Only	80%
Low	High	$500 per I/P Admit, $10 per Visit	Unmanaged Care	100%
High	Low	$500 per I/P Admit, $10 per Visit	Aggressively Managed Care, Inpatient Only	100%
National	High	$500 per I/P Admit, $10 per Visit	Moderately Managed Care, Inpatient and Outpatient	100%
National	National	$500 per I/P Admit, $10 per Visit	Unmanaged Care	80%
High	National	$250 per I/P Admit, $5 per Visit	Moderately Managed Care, Inpatient and Outpatient	80%
National	High	None	Moderately Managed Care, Inpatient and Outpatient	90%
Low	High	None	Unmanaged Care	90%
National	High	$250 per I/P Admit, $5 per Visit	Aggressively Managed Care, Inpatient Only	100%

No explicit margins or allowances for administrative expenses, coordination of benefits, stop loss reinsurance, adverse risks, or margins for profits and/or contingencies beyond those implicitly provided within the average costs per unit of service have been used.

Appendix III
Medicare Population Capitation Rates Sorted by Scenario Rate
PMPM Capitation Payments by Scenario
Estimated Psych & Substance Abuse Costs as of July 1, 1995

Utilization Level	Cost Level	Copay Level	Management Type	% of Medicare Allowable
Capitation at least $4.25 but less than $4.50				
National	National	None	Moderately Managed Care, Inpatient and Outpatient	100%
High	Low	$250 per I/P Admit, $5 per Visit	Moderately Managed Care, Inpatient and Outpatient	90%
National	National	$250 per I/P Admit, $5 per Visit	Moderately Managed Care, Inpatient Only	90%
Low	National	None	Unmanaged Care	100%
National	High	$250 per I/P Admit, $5 per Visit	Moderately Managed Care, Inpatient Only	80%
National	Low	$500 per I/P Admit, $10 per Visit	Unmanaged Care	90%
High	Low	$250 per I/P Admit, $5 per Visit	Aggressively Managed Care, Inpatient Only	90%
National	Low	None	Unmanaged Care	80%
High	National	$250 per I/P Admit, $5 per Visit	Aggressively Managed Care, Inpatient Only	80%
High	Low	$500 per I/P Admit, $10 per Visit	Moderately Managed Care, Inpatient Only	80%
National	Low	$250 per I/P Admit, $5 per Visit	Moderately Managed Care, Inpatient Only	100%
High	High	None	Aggressively Managed Care, Inpatient and Outpatient	100%
Low	High	None	Moderately Managed Care, Inpatient Only	100%
National	High	$250 per I/P Admit, $5 per Visit	Moderately Managed Care, Inpatient and Outpatient	90%
High	National	$500 per I/P Admit, $10 per Visit	Moderately Managed Care, Inpatient and Outpatient	80%
National	National	None	Aggressively Managed Care, Inpatient Only	100%
Low	High	$250 per I/P Admit, $5 per Visit	Unmanaged Care	90%
National	High	None	Aggressively Managed Care, Inpatient Only	90%
National	Low	$500 per I/P Admit, $10 per Visit	Moderately Managed Care, Inpatient Only	80%
National	High	$500 per I/P Admit, $10 per Visit	Aggressively Managed Care, Inpatient Only	100%
National	National	$250 per I/P Admit, $5 per Visit	Moderately Managed Care, Inpatient and Outpatient	100%
National	High	$500 per I/P Admit, $10 per Visit	Moderately Managed Care, Inpatient Only	80%
Low	National	$250 per I/P Admit, $5 per Visit	Unmanaged Care	100%
Capitation at least $4.00 but less than $4.25				
National	National	$500 per I/P Admit, $10 per Visit	Moderately Managed Care, Inpatient Only	90%
High	Low	$500 per I/P Admit, $10 per Visit	Moderately Managed Care, Inpatient and Outpatient	90%
National	National	None	Moderately Managed Care, Inpatient Only	80%
High	Low	None	Aggressively Managed Care, Inpatient Only	80%
High	Low	None	Moderately Managed Care, Inpatient and Outpatient	80%
National	Low	$250 per I/P Admit, $5 per Visit	Unmanaged Care	80%
High	High	$250 per I/P Admit, $5 per Visit	Aggressively Managed Care, Inpatient and Outpatient	100%
National	Low	None	Moderately Managed Care, Inpatient Only	90%
Low	High	$250 per I/P Admit, $5 per Visit	Moderately Managed Care, Inpatient Only	100%
Low	High	$500 per I/P Admit, $10 per Visit	Unmanaged Care	90%
National	High	$500 per I/P Admit, $10 per Visit	Moderately Managed Care, Inpatient and Outpatient	90%
High	Low	$500 per I/P Admit, $10 per Visit	Aggressively Managed Care, Inpatient Only	90%
High	National	$500 per I/P Admit, $10 per Visit	Aggressively Managed Care, Inpatient Only	80%
National	Low	$500 per I/P Admit, $10 per Visit	Moderately Managed Care, Inpatient Only	100%
National	National	$250 per I/P Admit, $5 per Visit	Aggressively Managed Care, Inpatient Only	100%
National	High	$250 per I/P Admit, $5 per Visit	Aggressively Managed Care, Inpatient Only	90%
National	National	$500 per I/P Admit, $10 per Visit	Moderately Managed Care, Inpatient and Outpatient	100%
National	National	None	Moderately Managed Care, Inpatient and Outpatient	90%
Low	National	$500 per I/P Admit, $10 per Visit	Unmanaged Care	100%
National	High	None	Moderately Managed Care, Inpatient and Outpatient	80%
Low	High	None	Moderately Managed Care, Inpatient and Outpatient	100%
Low	High	None	Unmanaged Care	80%
Low	National	None	Unmanaged Care	90%
High	High	$500 per I/P Admit, $10 per Visit	Aggressively Managed Care, Inpatient and Outpatient	100%

No explicit margins or allowances for administrative expenses, coordination of benefits, stop loss reinsurance, adverse risks, or margins for profits and/or contingencies beyond those implicitly provided within the average costs per unit of service have been used.

Appendix III
Medicare Population Capitation Rates Sorted by Scenario Rate
PMPM Capitation Payments by Scenario
Estimated Psych & Substance Abuse Costs as of July 1, 1995

Utilization Level	Cost Level	Copay Level	Management Type	% of Medicare Allowable
Capitation at least $3.75 but less than $4.00				
National	National	$250 per I/P Admit, $5 per Visit	Moderately Managed Care, Inpatient Only	80%
High	Low	$250 per I/P Admit, $5 per Visit	Moderately Managed Care, Inpatient and Outpatient	80%
Low	High	$500 per I/P Admit, $10 per Visit	Moderately Managed Care, Inpatient Only	100%
National	Low	$500 per I/P Admit, $10 per Visit	Unmanaged Care	80%
High	Low	$250 per I/P Admit, $5 per Visit	Aggressively Managed Care, Inpatient Only	80%
National	Low	$250 per I/P Admit, $5 per Visit	Moderately Managed Care, Inpatient Only	90%
National	Low	None	Moderately Managed Care, Inpatient and Outpatient	100%
High	High	None	Aggressively Managed Care, Inpatient and Outpatient	90%
High	National	None	Aggressively Managed Care, Inpatient and Outpatient	100%
Low	High	None	Moderately Managed Care, Inpatient Only	90%
Low	National	None	Moderately Managed Care, Inpatient Only	100%
Low	Low	None	Unmanaged Care	100%
National	National	None	Aggressively Managed Care, Inpatient Only	90%
National	Low	None	Aggressively Managed Care, Inpatient Only	100%
National	High	$250 per I/P Admit, $5 per Visit	Moderately Managed Care, Inpatient and Outpatient	80%
Low	High	$250 per I/P Admit, $5 per Visit	Unmanaged Care	80%
Low	High	None	Aggressively Managed Care, Inpatient Only	100%
Low	High	$250 per I/P Admit, $5 per Visit	Moderately Managed Care, Inpatient and Outpatient	100%
National	High	$500 per I/P Admit, $10 per Visit	Aggressively Managed Care, Inpatient Only	90%
National	National	$500 per I/P Admit, $10 per Visit	Aggressively Managed Care, Inpatient Only	100%
National	National	$250 per I/P Admit, $5 per Visit	Moderately Managed Care, Inpatient and Outpatient	90%
Low	National	$250 per I/P Admit, $5 per Visit	Unmanaged Care	90%
National	High	None	Aggressively Managed Care, Inpatient Only	80%
National	National	$500 per I/P Admit, $10 per Visit	Moderately Managed Care, Inpatient Only	80%
High	High	$250 per I/P Admit, $5 per Visit	Aggressively Managed Care, Inpatient and Outpatient	90%
High	Low	$500 per I/P Admit, $10 per Visit	Moderately Managed Care, Inpatient and Outpatient	80%
Low	High	$250 per I/P Admit, $5 per Visit	Moderately Managed Care, Inpatient Only	90%
Capitation at least $3.50 but less than $3.75				
High	National	$250 per I/P Admit, $5 per Visit	Aggressively Managed Care, Inpatient and Outpatient	100%
National	Low	$250 per I/P Admit, $5 per Visit	Moderately Managed Care, Inpatient and Outpatient	100%
National	Low	None	Moderately Managed Care, Inpatient Only	80%
Low	National	$250 per I/P Admit, $5 per Visit	Moderately Managed Care, Inpatient Only	100%
National	High	$500 per I/P Admit, $10 per Visit	Moderately Managed Care, Inpatient and Outpatient	80%
High	Low	$500 per I/P Admit, $10 per Visit	Aggressively Managed Care, Inpatient Only	80%
Low	High	$500 per I/P Admit, $10 per Visit	Unmanaged Care	80%
National	Low	$500 per I/P Admit, $10 per Visit	Moderately Managed Care, Inpatient Only	90%
Low	High	$500 per I/P Admit, $10 per Visit	Moderately Managed Care, Inpatient and Outpatient	100%
National	National	$250 per I/P Admit, $5 per Visit	Aggressively Managed Care, Inpatient Only	90%
Low	Low	$250 per I/P Admit, $5 per Visit	Unmanaged Care	100%
Low	High	$250 per I/P Admit, $5 per Visit	Aggressively Managed Care, Inpatient Only	100%
National	Low	$250 per I/P Admit, $5 per Visit	Aggressively Managed Care, Inpatient Only	100%
National	National	$500 per I/P Admit, $10 per Visit	Moderately Managed Care, Inpatient and Outpatient	90%
Low	National	$500 per I/P Admit, $10 per Visit	Unmanaged Care	90%
Low	High	None	Moderately Managed Care, Inpatient and Outpatient	90%
National	High	$250 per I/P Admit, $5 per Visit	Aggressively Managed Care, Inpatient Only	80%
High	High	$500 per I/P Admit, $10 per Visit	Aggressively Managed Care, Inpatient and Outpatient	90%
National	National	None	Moderately Managed Care, Inpatient and Outpatient	80%
Low	National	None	Moderately Managed Care, Inpatient and Outpatient	100%
Low	National	None	Unmanaged Care	80%
Low	High	$500 per I/P Admit, $10 per Visit	Moderately Managed Care, Inpatient Only	90%
High	National	$500 per I/P Admit, $10 per Visit	Aggressively Managed Care, Inpatient and Outpatient	100%
National	Low	None	Moderately Managed Care, Inpatient and Outpatient	90%
High	National	None	Aggressively Managed Care, Inpatient and Outpatient	90%
Low	National	None	Moderately Managed Care, Inpatient Only	90%
Low	National	$500 per I/P Admit, $10 per Visit	Moderately Managed Care, Inpatient Only	100%
National	Low	None	Aggressively Managed Care, Inpatient Only	90%
Low	Low	None	Unmanaged Care	90%
National	Low	$500 per I/P Admit, $10 per Visit	Moderately Managed Care, Inpatient and Outpatient	100%
High	High	None	Aggressively Managed Care, Inpatient and Outpatient	80%

No explicit margins or allowances for administrative expenses, coordination of benefits, stop loss reinsurance, adverse risks, or margins for profits and/or contingencies beyond those implicitly provided within the average costs per unit of service have been used.

Appendix III
Medicare Population Capitation Rates Sorted by Scenario Rate
PMPM Capitation Payments by Scenario
Estimated Psych & Substance Abuse Costs as of July 1, 1995

Utilization Level	Cost Level	Copay Level	Management Type	% of Medicare Allowable
Capitation at least $3.25 but less than $3.50				
National	Low	$250 per I/P Admit, $5 per Visit	Moderately Managed Care, Inpatient Only	80%
Low	High	None	Moderately Managed Care, Inpatient Only	80%
Low	High	$500 per I/P Admit, $10 per Visit	Aggressively Managed Care, Inpatient Only	100%
Low	High	$250 per I/P Admit, $5 per Visit	Moderately Managed Care, Inpatient and Outpatient	90%
Low	Low	$500 per I/P Admit, $10 per Visit	Unmanaged Care	100%
Low	National	None	Aggressively Managed Care, Inpatient Only	100%
Low	High	None	Aggressively Managed Care, Inpatient Only	90%
High	Low	None	Aggressively Managed Care, Inpatient and Outpatient	100%
National	National	None	Aggressively Managed Care, Inpatient Only	80%
National	National	$500 per I/P Admit, $10 per Visit	Aggressively Managed Care, Inpatient Only	90%
Low	Low	None	Moderately Managed Care, Inpatient Only	100%
National	National	$250 per I/P Admit, $5 per Visit	Moderately Managed Care, Inpatient and Outpatient	80%
National	High	$500 per I/P Admit, $10 per Visit	Aggressively Managed Care, Inpatient Only	80%
Low	National	$250 per I/P Admit, $5 per Visit	Moderately Managed Care, Inpatient and Outpatient	100%
National	Low	$500 per I/P Admit, $10 per Visit	Aggressively Managed Care, Inpatient Only	100%
Low	National	$250 per I/P Admit, $5 per Visit	Unmanaged Care	80%
High	National	$250 per I/P Admit, $5 per Visit	Aggressively Managed Care, Inpatient and Outpatient	90%
National	Low	$250 per I/P Admit, $5 per Visit	Moderately Managed Care, Inpatient and Outpatient	90%
High	High	$250 per I/P Admit, $5 per Visit	Aggressively Managed Care, Inpatient and Outpatient	80%
Low	High	$250 per I/P Admit, $5 per Visit	Moderately Managed Care, Inpatient Only	80%
Low	National	$250 per I/P Admit, $5 per Visit	Moderately Managed Care, Inpatient Only	90%
Low	High	$500 per I/P Admit, $10 per Visit	Moderately Managed Care, Inpatient and Outpatient	90%
Low	Low	$250 per I/P Admit, $5 per Visit	Unmanaged Care	90%
Low	High	$250 per I/P Admit, $5 per Visit	Aggressively Managed Care, Inpatient Only	90%
National	Low	$250 per I/P Admit, $5 per Visit	Aggressively Managed Care, Inpatient Only	90%
High	Low	$250 per I/P Admit, $5 per Visit	Aggressively Managed Care, Inpatient and Outpatient	100%
Low	National	$250 per I/P Admit, $5 per Visit	Aggressively Managed Care, Inpatient Only	100%
National	National	$250 per I/P Admit, $5 per Visit	Aggressively Managed Care, Inpatient Only	80%
National	High	None	Aggressively Managed Care, Inpatient and Outpatient	100%
Low	High	None	Aggressively Managed Care, Inpatient and Outpatient	100%
National	National	$500 per I/P Admit, $10 per Visit	Moderately Managed Care, Inpatient and Outpatient	80%

No explicit margins or allowances for administrative expenses, coordination of benefits, stop loss reinsurance, adverse risks, or margins for profits and/or contingencies beyond those implicitly provided within the average costs per unit of service have been used.

Appendix III
Medicare Population Capitation Rates Sorted by Scenario Rate
PMPM Capitation Payments by Scenario
Estimated Psych & Substance Abuse Costs as of July 1, 1995

Utilization Level	Cost Level	Copay Level	Management Type	% of Medicare Allowable
Capitation at least $3.00 but less than $3.25				
Low	Low	$250 per I/P Admit, $5 per Visit	Moderately Managed Care, Inpatient Only	100%
Low	National	$500 per I/P Admit, $10 per Visit	Moderately Managed Care, Inpatient and Outpatient	100%
Low	National	None	Moderately Managed Care, Inpatient and Outpatient	90%
Low	National	$500 per I/P Admit, $10 per Visit	Unmanaged Care	80%
Low	High	None	Moderately Managed Care, Inpatient and Outpatient	80%
High	High	$500 per I/P Admit, $10 per Visit	Aggressively Managed Care, Inpatient and Outpatient	80%
High	National	$500 per I/P Admit, $10 per Visit	Aggressively Managed Care, Inpatient and Outpatient	90%
Low	High	$500 per I/P Admit, $10 per Visit	Moderately Managed Care, Inpatient Only	80%
Low	Low	None	Moderately Managed Care, Inpatient and Outpatient	100%
National	Low	$500 per I/P Admit, $10 per Visit	Moderately Managed Care, Inpatient and Outpatient	90%
National	Low	None	Moderately Managed Care, Inpatient and Outpatient	80%
Low	National	$500 per I/P Admit, $10 per Visit	Moderately Managed Care, Inpatient Only	90%
Low	High	$500 per I/P Admit, $10 per Visit	Aggressively Managed Care, Inpatient Only	90%
High	National	None	Aggressively Managed Care, Inpatient and Outpatient	80%
Low	High	$250 per I/P Admit, $5 per Visit	Aggressively Managed Care, Inpatient and Outpatient	100%
High	Low	None	Aggressively Managed Care, Inpatient and Outpatient	90%
Low	National	None	Aggressively Managed Care, Inpatient Only	90%
National	High	$250 per I/P Admit, $5 per Visit	Aggressively Managed Care, Inpatient and Outpatient	100%
Low	National	None	Moderately Managed Care, Inpatient Only	80%
Low	Low	$500 per I/P Admit, $10 per Visit	Unmanaged Care	90%
Low	Low	None	Unmanaged Care	80%
National	Low	None	Aggressively Managed Care, Inpatient Only	80%
Low	National	$500 per I/P Admit, $10 per Visit	Aggressively Managed Care, Inpatient Only	100%
High	Low	$500 per I/P Admit, $10 per Visit	Aggressively Managed Care, Inpatient and Outpatient	100%
Low	Low	None	Moderately Managed Care, Inpatient Only	90%
Low	Low	None	Aggressively Managed Care, Inpatient Only	100%
Low	High	$250 per I/P Admit, $5 per Visit	Moderately Managed Care, Inpatient and Outpatient	80%
Low	High	None	Aggressively Managed Care, Inpatient Only	80%
Low	National	$250 per I/P Admit, $5 per Visit	Moderately Managed Care, Inpatient and Outpatient	90%
National	National	$500 per I/P Admit, $10 per Visit	Aggressively Managed Care, Inpatient Only	80%
National	Low	$500 per I/P Admit, $10 per Visit	Aggressively Managed Care, Inpatient Only	90%
Low	Low	$500 per I/P Admit, $10 per Visit	Moderately Managed Care, Inpatient Only	100%

No explicit margins or allowances for administrative expenses, coordination of benefits, stop loss reinsurance, adverse risks, or margins for profits and/or contingencies beyond those implicitly provided within the average costs per unit of service have been used.

Appendix III
Medicare Population Capitation Rates Sorted by Scenario Rate
PMPM Capitation Payments by Scenario
Estimated Psych & Substance Abuse Costs as of July 1, 1995

Utilization Level	Cost Level	Copay Level	Management Type	% of Medicare Allowable
Capitation at least $2.75 but less than $3.00				
High	National	$250 per I/P Admit, $5 per Visit	Aggressively Managed Care, Inpatient and Outpatient	80%
National	High	$500 per I/P Admit, $10 per Visit	Aggressively Managed Care, Inpatient and Outpatient	100%
Low	Low	$250 per I/P Admit, $5 per Visit	Moderately Managed Care, Inpatient and Outpatient	100%
Low	High	$500 per I/P Admit, $10 per Visit	Aggressively Managed Care, Inpatient and Outpatient	100%
National	Low	$250 per I/P Admit, $5 per Visit	Moderately Managed Care, Inpatient and Outpatient	80%
Low	National	$250 per I/P Admit, $5 per Visit	Moderately Managed Care, Inpatient Only	80%
Low	National	$250 per I/P Admit, $5 per Visit	Aggressively Managed Care, Inpatient Only	90%
High	Low	$250 per I/P Admit, $5 per Visit	Aggressively Managed Care, Inpatient and Outpatient	90%
Low	Low	$250 per I/P Admit, $5 per Visit	Unmanaged Care	80%
Low	High	None	Aggressively Managed Care, Inpatient and Outpatient	90%
Low	High	$500 per I/P Admit, $10 per Visit	Moderately Managed Care, Inpatient and Outpatient	80%
National	High	None	Aggressively Managed Care, Inpatient and Outpatient	90%
Low	National	None	Aggressively Managed Care, Inpatient and Outpatient	100%
Low	High	$250 per I/P Admit, $5 per Visit	Aggressively Managed Care, Inpatient Only	80%
National	National	None	Aggressively Managed Care, Inpatient and Outpatient	100%
National	Low	$250 per I/P Admit, $5 per Visit	Aggressively Managed Care, Inpatient Only	80%
Low	Low	$250 per I/P Admit, $5 per Visit	Moderately Managed Care, Inpatient Only	90%
Low	National	$500 per I/P Admit, $10 per Visit	Moderately Managed Care, Inpatient and Outpatient	90%
Low	Low	$250 per I/P Admit, $5 per Visit	Aggressively Managed Care, Inpatient Only	100%
Low	National	None	Moderately Managed Care, Inpatient and Outpatient	80%
Low	Low	None	Moderately Managed Care, Inpatient and Outpatient	90%
High	National	$500 per I/P Admit, $10 per Visit	Aggressively Managed Care, Inpatient and Outpatient	80%
National	High	$250 per I/P Admit, $5 per Visit	Aggressively Managed Care, Inpatient and Outpatient	90%
Low	High	$250 per I/P Admit, $5 per Visit	Aggressively Managed Care, Inpatient and Outpatient	90%
Low	National	$500 per I/P Admit, $10 per Visit	Moderately Managed Care, Inpatient Only	80%
National	Low	$500 per I/P Admit, $10 per Visit	Moderately Managed Care, Inpatient and Outpatient	80%
Low	National	$500 per I/P Admit, $10 per Visit	Aggressively Managed Care, Inpatient Only	90%
Low	Low	$500 per I/P Admit, $10 per Visit	Moderately Managed Care, Inpatient and Outpatient	100%
National	National	$250 per I/P Admit, $5 per Visit	Aggressively Managed Care, Inpatient and Outpatient	100%
Low	Low	$500 per I/P Admit, $10 per Visit	Unmanaged Care	80%
Low	National	None	Aggressively Managed Care, Inpatient Only	80%
Low	Low	None	Aggressively Managed Care, Inpatient Only	90%
High	Low	$500 per I/P Admit, $10 per Visit	Aggressively Managed Care, Inpatient and Outpatient	90%
Low	National	$250 per I/P Admit, $5 per Visit	Aggressively Managed Care, Inpatient and Outpatient	100%
Low	High	$500 per I/P Admit, $10 per Visit	Aggressively Managed Care, Inpatient Only	80%
High	Low	None	Aggressively Managed Care, Inpatient and Outpatient	80%
Low	Low	None	Moderately Managed Care, Inpatient Only	80%

No explicit margins or allowances for administrative expenses, coordination of benefits, stop loss reinsurance, adverse risks, or margins for profits and/or contingencies beyond those implicitly provided within the average costs per unit of service have been used.

Appendix III
Medicare Population Capitation Rates Sorted by Scenario Rate
PMPM Capitation Payments by Scenario
Estimated Psych & Substance Abuse Costs as of July 1, 1995

Utilization Level	Cost Level	Copay Level	Management Type	% of Medicare Allowable
Capitation at least $2.50 but less than $2.75				
Low	Low	$500 per I/P Admit, $10 per Visit	Moderately Managed Care, Inpatient Only	90%
Low	National	$250 per I/P Admit, $5 per Visit	Moderately Managed Care, Inpatient and Outpatient	80%
Low	Low	$500 per I/P Admit, $10 per Visit	Aggressively Managed Care, Inpatient Only	100%
National	Low	$500 per I/P Admit, $10 per Visit	Aggressively Managed Care, Inpatient Only	80%
National	High	$500 per I/P Admit, $10 per Visit	Aggressively Managed Care, Inpatient and Outpatient	90%
Low	High	$500 per I/P Admit, $10 per Visit	Aggressively Managed Care, Inpatient and Outpatient	90%
Low	Low	$250 per I/P Admit, $5 per Visit	Moderately Managed Care, Inpatient and Outpatient	90%
Low	National	$250 per I/P Admit, $5 per Visit	Aggressively Managed Care, Inpatient Only	80%
Low	National	$500 per I/P Admit, $10 per Visit	Aggressively Managed Care, Inpatient and Outpatient	100%
National	National	None	Aggressively Managed Care, Inpatient and Outpatient	90%
Low	National	None	Aggressively Managed Care, Inpatient and Outpatient	90%
National	National	$500 per I/P Admit, $10 per Visit	Aggressively Managed Care, Inpatient and Outpatient	100%
High	Low	$250 per I/P Admit, $5 per Visit	Aggressively Managed Care, Inpatient and Outpatient	80%
Low	Low	$250 per I/P Admit, $5 per Visit	Aggressively Managed Care, Inpatient Only	90%
National	High	None	Aggressively Managed Care, Inpatient and Outpatient	80%
Low	High	None	Aggressively Managed Care, Inpatient and Outpatient	80%
Low	Low	$250 per I/P Admit, $5 per Visit	Moderately Managed Care, Inpatient Only	80%
Low	National	$500 per I/P Admit, $10 per Visit	Moderately Managed Care, Inpatient and Outpatient	80%
National	Low	None	Aggressively Managed Care, Inpatient and Outpatient	100%
Low	Low	None	Aggressively Managed Care, Inpatient and Outpatient	100%
Low	Low	None	Moderately Managed Care, Inpatient and Outpatient	80%
Low	Low	$500 per I/P Admit, $10 per Visit	Moderately Managed Care, Inpatient and Outpatient	90%
Low	National	$250 per I/P Admit, $5 per Visit	Aggressively Managed Care, Inpatient and Outpatient	90%
National	National	$250 per I/P Admit, $5 per Visit	Aggressively Managed Care, Inpatient and Outpatient	90%
National	High	$250 per I/P Admit, $5 per Visit	Aggressively Managed Care, Inpatient and Outpatient	80%
Low	High	$250 per I/P Admit, $5 per Visit	Aggressively Managed Care, Inpatient and Outpatient	80%
Capitation at least $2.25 but less than $2.50				
Low	National	$500 per I/P Admit, $10 per Visit	Aggressively Managed Care, Inpatient Only	80%
High	Low	$500 per I/P Admit, $10 per Visit	Aggressively Managed Care, Inpatient and Outpatient	80%
Low	Low	None	Aggressively Managed Care, Inpatient Only	80%
Low	Low	$500 per I/P Admit, $10 per Visit	Aggressively Managed Care, Inpatient Only	90%
Low	Low	$500 per I/P Admit, $10 per Visit	Moderately Managed Care, Inpatient Only	80%
National	Low	$250 per I/P Admit, $5 per Visit	Aggressively Managed Care, Inpatient and Outpatient	100%
Low	Low	$250 per I/P Admit, $5 per Visit	Aggressively Managed Care, Inpatient and Outpatient	100%
Low	Low	$250 per I/P Admit, $5 per Visit	Moderately Managed Care, Inpatient and Outpatient	80%
Low	High	$500 per I/P Admit, $10 per Visit	Aggressively Managed Care, Inpatient and Outpatient	80%
National	High	$500 per I/P Admit, $10 per Visit	Aggressively Managed Care, Inpatient and Outpatient	80%
National	National	$500 per I/P Admit, $10 per Visit	Aggressively Managed Care, Inpatient and Outpatient	90%
Low	National	$500 per I/P Admit, $10 per Visit	Aggressively Managed Care, Inpatient and Outpatient	90%
National	National	None	Aggressively Managed Care, Inpatient and Outpatient	80%
Low	National	None	Aggressively Managed Care, Inpatient and Outpatient	80%
National	Low	None	Aggressively Managed Care, Inpatient and Outpatient	90%
Low	Low	None	Aggressively Managed Care, Inpatient and Outpatient	90%
Low	Low	$250 per I/P Admit, $5 per Visit	Aggressively Managed Care, Inpatient Only	80%
National	Low	$500 per I/P Admit, $10 per Visit	Aggressively Managed Care, Inpatient and Outpatient	100%
Low	Low	$500 per I/P Admit, $10 per Visit	Aggressively Managed Care, Inpatient and Outpatient	100%

No explicit margins or allowances for administrative expenses, coordination of benefits, stop loss reinsurance, adverse risks, or margins for profits and/or contingencies beyond those implicitly provided within the average costs per unit of service have been used.

Appendix III
Medicare Population Capitation Rates Sorted by Scenario Rate
PMPM Capitation Payments by Scenario
Estimated Psych & Substance Abuse Costs as of July 1, 1995

Utilization Level	Cost Level	Copay Level	Management Type	% of Medicare Allowable
Capitation at least $2.00 but less than $2.25				
Low	Low	$500 per I/P Admit, $10 per Visit	Moderately Managed Care, Inpatient and Outpatient	80%
Low	National	$250 per I/P Admit, $5 per Visit	Aggressively Managed Care, Inpatient and Outpatient	80%
National	National	$250 per I/P Admit, $5 per Visit	Aggressively Managed Care, Inpatient and Outpatient	80%
Low	Low	$250 per I/P Admit, $5 per Visit	Aggressively Managed Care, Inpatient and Outpatient	90%
National	Low	$250 per I/P Admit, $5 per Visit	Aggressively Managed Care, Inpatient and Outpatient	90%
Low	Low	$500 per I/P Admit, $10 per Visit	Aggressively Managed Care, Inpatient Only	80%
Low	National	$500 per I/P Admit, $10 per Visit	Aggressively Managed Care, Inpatient and Outpatient	80%
National	National	$500 per I/P Admit, $10 per Visit	Aggressively Managed Care, Inpatient and Outpatient	80%
National	Low	None	Aggressively Managed Care, Inpatient and Outpatient	80%
Low	Low	None	Aggressively Managed Care, Inpatient and Outpatient	80%
National	Low	$500 per I/P Admit, $10 per Visit	Aggressively Managed Care, Inpatient and Outpatient	90%
Low	Low	$500 per I/P Admit, $10 per Visit	Aggressively Managed Care, Inpatient and Outpatient	90%
Capitation at least $1.75 but less than $2.00				
National	Low	$250 per I/P Admit, $5 per Visit	Aggressively Managed Care, Inpatient and Outpatient	80%
Low	Low	$250 per I/P Admit, $5 per Visit	Aggressively Managed Care, Inpatient and Outpatient	80%
National	Low	$500 per I/P Admit, $10 per Visit	Aggressively Managed Care, Inpatient and Outpatient	80%
Low	Low	$500 per I/P Admit, $10 per Visit	Aggressively Managed Care, Inpatient and Outpatient	80%

No explicit margins or allowances for administrative expenses, coordination of benefits, stop loss reinsurance, adverse risks, or margins for profits and/or contingencies beyond those implicitly provided within the average costs per unit of service have been used.

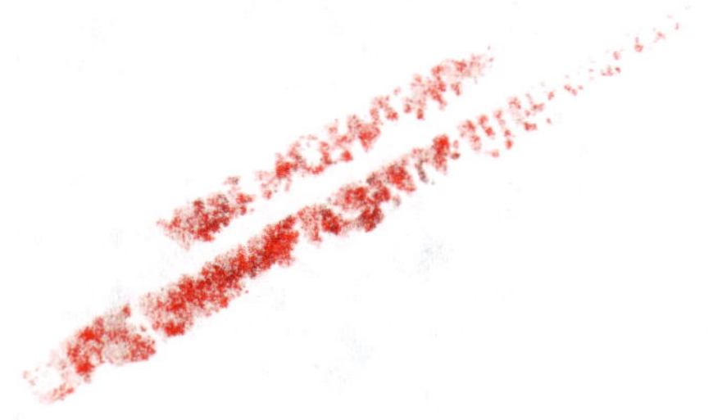